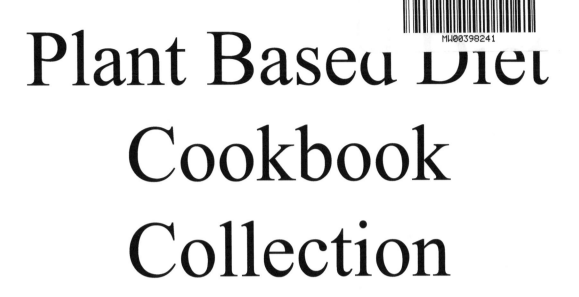

Plant Based Diet Cookbook Collection

Plant Based Breakfasts, Lunches, and Dinners Plus Appetizers and Desserts

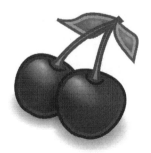

Bindi Wetzel

Plant Based Diet Cookbook Collection

Published by United Publishing House

ISBN-13: 978-1492715641
ISBN-10:1492715646

www.UnitedPublishingHouse.com
Email: Authors@UnitedPublishingHouse.com

Printed in U.S.A

Table of Contents

Other Books by Bindi Wetzel

Plant Based Nutrition: A Quick Start Guide for a Plant Based Diet

Plant Based Breakfast Recipes

Plant Based Lunch Recipes

Plant Based Dinner Recipes

Healthy Vegetarian Breakfasts

Healthy Vegetarian Lunches

Healthy Vegetarian Dinners

Healthy Vegetarian Collection

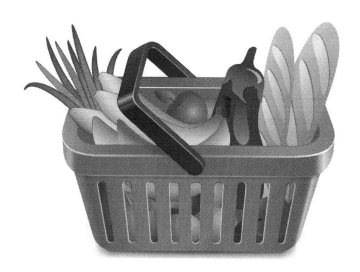

A Glimpse at Plant-Based Eating

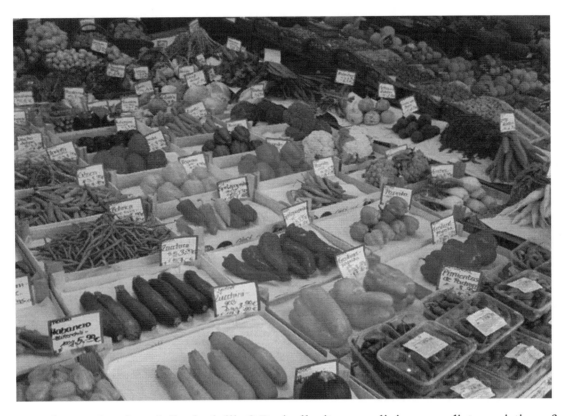

What does a plant based diet look like? Basically, it means living on a diet consisting of grains, nuts, seeds, meat and cheese substitutes, fruits and vegetables that are seasonal and of the highest quality you can afford. Some of the foods you will regularly find in a plant-based diet are:

- Vegetables of every kind

- All kinds of fruits

- Grains (non-genetically engineered foods), rices and cereals

- All seeds and nuts

- Meat and cheese substitutes

- Nut milks and butters

- Herbs and spices

- Vinegars and oils

There are many different reasons why someone would choose to eat a plant-based diet. For me, it was a way of life growing up. It has always been the way I've eaten and I've never felt like I have missed out because I don't eat meat. I thoroughly enjoy eating a plant-based diet and invite you to join me. Below are a few points on why many others choose to eat this way.

1. Some plant-based eaters condemn meat eating due to the nature of the way animals are killed for food. Many believe meat is not needed in the human diet for survival and is not necessary to remain healthy. They believe animals have as much of a right to live as humans do.

2. Some are interested in cutting down on the fat in their diet. While meats do provide a lot of protein, they also include fat. Therefore, the reasoning is, if you cut out meat, you will be cutting out fats as well – some are good while others are bad. By cutting out both kinds of fat, bad ones can be replaced with foods that are lower in fat and contain good ones.

3. Some desire to cut out meats from their diet to help with weight loss. Eliminating meat can be done wisely if you do not turn to unhealthy foods like French fries, chips, and veggie pizzas exclusively. You have to eat smart by eating more of healthy vegetables and fruits.

4. Some people become plant based eaters simply because they believe it is a healthier way to eat. Replacing meat with more foods like fruits, beans, whole grains, and vegetables can certainly lead to getting more nutrients your body needs, resulting in better health, experiencing more energy, and being ill less often than you used to be.

5. Since the publication of *The China Study* and the work of Caldwell Esselstyn, many believe there is a direct link between cancer rates and meat consumption. This study advocates that by eliminating meat from your diet, becoming a plant-based eater can result in heart disease being reversed and damaged arteries being repaired.

Types of Plant-Based Eaters

For some, becoming a plant-based eater is a snap decision. For others, it is a process with many steps along the way. It may surprise you to find that there are numerous types of plant-based eaters.

I thought I would take a few sentences to tell you about a few because if you are exploring this lifestyle, you may find you have more choices than you realized in your journey toward plant-based eating.

- Vegetarianism ~ This plant-based diet is one that can include cheese, milk and eggs if desired

- Semi-vegetarianism ~ This form of eating allows occasional meat products. A new term called "Flexitarians" has become a way to label vegetarians who occasionally enjoy meat. This step is between a meat-eater and a plant-eater which may make it easier for you while you are transitioning. At the same time, you may decide you want to remain a flexitarian. If so, this is perfectly fine, too. Many find this compromise works great for them because it allows flexibility, especially when eating with others outside their home and in situations related to their businesses.

- Other types of "semi-vegetarians" are "Pescetarians" who eat fish while "Pollotarians" eat fowl and poultry. Yet, there are also "Pese-Pollotarians" who consume poultry and fish but refuse to eat any red meat.

- Nutritarian ~ This diet described people who consume calories with as many micronutrients in them as possible while eating mostly vegetables and fruits with no processed foods

- Veganism ~ This plant-based diet does not allow any animal food sources. "Raw veganism" refers to vegans that consume foods that are uncooked or dehydrated while "Fruitarians" are vegans who mostly consumes fruit

- Macrobiotic diet ~ This plant-based diet is mostly vegetarian with some occasional consumption of seafood

As you can see, there are several steps and layers involved in a plant-based diet and you may find yourself wearing several different "labels" before you finally settle into an eating style you are comfortable with. Just remember, this is a journey toward a lifestyle where you may encounter several twists and turns along the way.

Support for Plant-Based Eating

More and more doctors are waking up to the fact that drugs and surgery do not effectively treat most degenerative diseases – much less prevent it. When they take a hard look at what the science says about diet and health, more and more of them are supporting healthy eating centered on unrefined plant foods.

The results of the 2011 research study conducted by Doctor Neal D. Barnard, M.D. found "people not only slim down, but also see their cholesterol levels plummet and their blood pressure fall. If they have diabetes, it typically improves and sometimes even disappears.

Arthritis pains and migraines often vanish, and energy comes racing back. Sluggishness vanishes, and they look and feel radiant."

According to the American Dietetic Association (ADA), "well-planned vegetarian diets are appropriate for individuals during all stages of the life-cycle, including pregnancy, lactation, infancy, childhood and adolescence and for athletes."

Plant based diets are often associated with health advantages including lower blood cholesterol levels, lower risk of heart disease, lower blood pressure levels and lower risk of hypertension and Type 2 diabetes, according to ADA's position.

The American Dietetic Association is the world's largest organization of food and nutrition professionals. ADA is committed to improving the nation's health and advancing the profession of dietetics through research, education and advocacy. Visit the American Dietetic Association at http://www.eatright.org for more information.

Things to Consider When Becoming a Plant-Based Eater

Here are some things to consider as you transition your way of eating as you change over to being a plant-based eater:

- Make sure you have good reasons for wanting to change to this way of eating. If you want to do this because you want to be part of the latest "fad" or because all your friends are doing it, you probably will not stick with it for very long. Becoming a plant-based eater is not a hard thing to do, but it is a lifestyle change and one that requires you to change your habits. You will need to be motivated to change so be sure to think this through carefully. Once you are convinced you should do it and really believe in what you want to do, the rest is easy.

- Don't get frustrated if you aren't able to make the transition to a meatless way of eating overnight. Start gradually. Begin by making simple substitutions in your favorite recipes. Many meat substitutes on the market are very good that you can try the next time you want a hamburger. Just make it a veggie burger instead.

- Read as much as you can about a plant-based diet. Know what areas you will need to focus on and foods you will need to include more often as you substitute other foods to obtain the proteins you will need.

- Make a list of the foods you are used to eating throughout a day and a week. Consider meat, poultry, and seafood. Go to the store and look in the freezer section. See what products are for sale that could be used as substitutes. Buy a few and try them the next time you want to make stir-fry. Try tofu instead of chicken. Try seitan instead of beef. You will be amazed at how many choices there are.

- Create a shopping list for your staples and foods you wish to keep on hand. Having food items and brand names listed on paper or in your phone make it helpful when you go shopping.

- Look for ethnic grocery stores, too. Many different cultures eat as plant eaters so this is a great time to discover new recipes, spices, and ingredients from other countries.

- Stay focused on your objective. Remember, you are trying to consider ways to eliminate meats in a healthy way. This does not mean eating a bunch of junk food. Focus more heavily on vegetables, fruits, beans, nuts, whole grains, and low-fat dairy products. Remember, you are talking about making a lifestyle change to get healthier so junk food should remain limited.

- Take time to plan your meals. Being able to eat healthy does require purchasing healthy food to have one hand. Keep healthy snacks with you for time when you are running errands. If you know you are going to a party, offer to bring a vegetarian dish. It helps the hostess and it certainly helps you.

- When you prepare your meals, make double and triple batches. Leftover can really come in handy when you don't feel like cooking or you had a very busy day and you didn't get a chance to prepare dinner ahead of time. Plus, leftovers make great lunches at home or at the office.

- Share with family and friends what you are doing. Don't get defensive and argumentative with others. Just explain what you are doing and why.

- Don't create a diet full of processed, sugary, white flour items just because you are eliminating meats. Choose wisely and pay attention to calories, fats, proteins, and fibers in your foods. Also choose the healthiest sources of food you can afford.

- Most of all, have fun. Do not think of a plant based way of eating as one that is restrictive. Consider it as a new adventure – one that will bring new things to discover and try as you look for great recipes to make and new foods to try.

Here is a simple plan many of my friends have used as they make the transition to plant-based eating:

1. Pick a date to begin to start making permanent changes in your diet

2. Pick one meal during this first week where you decide to eliminate meat from a meal you would normally have

3. Now choose a date in the next week where you decide to eliminate meat from another meal

4. Now make a decision to totally eliminate one kind of meat from your diet completely

5. For the next week, make a decision to eliminate another kind of meat from your diet

Next, address the issue of dairy products if you decide you need, or want to:

1. Pick a day during the week where you will have a dairy-free meal that normally would include it. Feel free to include dairy substitutes here

2. In the next week, pick another meal where there is no dairy included

3. Make a decision to totally eliminate one type of dairy from your diet

4. In the next week, decide to remove another dairy item from your diet

5. Continue until you have eliminated dairy completely

Finally, the last step is eliminating eggs from your diet

1. Choose a meal that would normally include eggs and make it without them. Egg substitutes are 99% egg whites so if you are trying to eliminate eggs, this is not how you do it. This means scrambled eggs will be difficult to imitate.

2. Eggs can be substituted in recipes by using items like baking powder combined with vinegar, apricot puree, or gelatin mixed with water.

As you eliminate meats and possibly dairy and eggs, it will be necessary for you to decide:

• What will you substitute in their place? Will you now use nut milks, meat substitutes (and which ones), and dairy alternatives?

• How will you incorporate whole and unprocessed foods into your diet?

• What do plant-based recipes look like for you? (I personally would recommend trying to pick a week's worth of menus with a shopping list and stick with these recipes until you are comfortable with your new style of eating, cooking, and shopping.)

My friends who have made the transition to plant-based eating have found it helpful to keep track of new foods, progress, difficulties, and even favorite recipes in a notebook, on their computers or phones as they make changes. I certainly would recommend you consider doing the same until you are comfortable with the challenges and changes of this lifestyle.

Healthy Changes for Becoming a Plant-Based Eater

As a plant eater, I have found myself making subtle changes as I have discovered healthier ways of eating. I wanted to share four specific areas you will have to deal with as you make this journey. These involve dealing with dairy, sugars, eggs, and meats.

1. DAIRY

Personally, I do not have any problems using or consuming dairy products in my diet. I do not have any allergies or intolerances with dairy, and like others who eat this way, I enjoy cheeses, yogurts, milk and creams. However, as I have researched and learned ways to eat healthier, I have been using various dairy alternatives in my cooking.

- Over time, I have been using more coconut and almond milk in my recipes. In addition, I try to use more cheeses that are aged when I cook or whenever I want a snack because the lactose levels almost disappear when cheeses are aged. This means the cheeses will not affect my blood sugar levels as dramatically as regular cheeses can. There are even some delicious cheeses and frozen desserts made with coconut, rice, and soy.

- Try experimenting with soy milk, soy-based cheeses and yogurts. Like me, I think you will find some incredibly appetizing choices that are delicious and good for you.

- Many of the recipes included in this collection do not include dairy and cheese, and remember you can substitute with dairy and cheese alternatives if you want to.

2. NATURAL SUGARS

Something I started doing years ago was learning more about natural sugars and how to use them in my cooking. Some can be substituted for granulated (white) sugar 1-for-1 while others cannot. Whenever possible, try to use organic, raw and natural sugars like those listed below in your recipes whenever it calls for sugar.

- Raw honey: not heated, strained, or filtered. High in B and C vitamins

- Coconut palm sugar: contains many minerals compared to white and brown sugar and doesn't raise your blood sugar levels very much

- Blackstrap molasses: high iron content and doesn't raise your blood sugar levels very much

- Sucanat: unrefined, whole cane sugar

- Pure maple syrup: Grade A is sweeter; not as strong as Grade B

- Stevia: calorie-free; comes in several forms

3. EGGS

If you are striving to eat as a vegan, eliminating eggs from your diet can be a challenge. Here are some suggestions to try in your recipes as you learn to make substitutions:

- Canned pumpkin ~ You can substitute ¼ cup of pumpkin for each egg called for in your recipe. This will only work with baked goods. Because you will be able to taste the pumpkin, consider using it in recipes that include ingredients like chocolate, cinnamon, carrots, and apples.

- Ener-G Egg Replacer® ~ For baked goods, you use 1½ teaspoons of powder with 2 teaspoons of water for each egg you are replacing.

- Applesauce ~ Use ¼ cup of applesauce to replace each egg in your baking recipes. It is great in pancakes and muffins.

- Nut and soy milks ~ Use one cup of milk to replace eggs used in recipes like French toast.

- Ground flaxseed ~ Use 1 tablespoon of ground flaxseed with 3 tablespoons of water for each egg being substituted. Stir until it becomes like a gelatin. This binds the ingredients together in your baked goods while adding moisture.

- Mashed banana ~ For each egg you want to replace, use ½ mashed banana in your baked goods. Works best in quick breads and muffins. Great for adding moisture to your foods.

4. MEATS

For some, eliminating meat from their diet so they can become plant eaters may be a challenge. However, it may be easier than you think. Meat substitutes that are plant based are so much better tasting than the early days of the initial veggie burgers. There are now meat substitutes that are made from wheat protein and soy and can be purchased frozen, dried or even fresh.

Here is a list of some options:

- Seitan ~ This great source of protein is derived from wheat. It is used as a substitute for chicken, roasts, and can be cooked and made into crumbles to sprinkle over pizzas and as ground beef.

- Tofu ~ Made from curdled soybean milk and water, tofu is high in calcium and protein and tends to take on flavors when marinades and spices are used. It is available in various forms: fresh, water-packed tofu which must always be refrigerated – used for grilling and baking; silken tofu that does not need refrigerated – usually used for desserts, creamy sauces and dressings; firm and extra-firm tofu – used for frying, grilling, sautéing and baking.

- Tempeh ~ Unlike tofu, tempeh is denser because it is has whole soybeans in it as well as other grains. Because of its denseness, it is usually good to simmer it in a flavored liquid to soften it.

5. NON-STICK COOKING SPRAYS

Non-stick cooking sprays usually contain propellants like isobutene, carbon dioxide and nitrogen dioxide and are ingredients I don't want to use in my cooking. Instead, you can do as I do and use a cooking spray bottle made for spraying oil. (Pampered Chef® and Misto Olive Oil Sprayer® are a couple you can choose from). You can fill them using 3 parts extra virgin olive oil to 5 parts water and shake each time before applying or just use straight olive oil. Then keep the bottle in the refrigerator to use whenever you need some and make more when you run out.

Please note: Throughout my cookbook I use the phrase, "non-stick cooking spray" when there is a need for applying something to help keep foods from sticking. However, I strongly suggest apply coconut oil using a paper towel or applying your own olive oil from a spray bottle. Plus, you still have the option of using a commercial cooking spray if you desire.

As you attempt some of the recipes in this collection, try incorporating some of the ideas I presented above to make substitutions in recipes that include ingredients you are trying not to eat. Most of them are highly adaptable for whatever kind of plant-based eater you are trying to be.

I think you will enjoy the results you get—not only in taste but just in knowing it is a healthy way to eat. Remember: experiment and have fun with the changes you are making. You have a lifetime to try new things.

A Plant-Based Grocery List

Depending upon where you are in your journey toward plant-based eating, shopping for foods you are not familiar with or may not have purchased before can prove expensive or leave you feeling uncertain. Below are some important points to consider as you begin to stock your pantry:

- The following list is a **guide**. It is *not* intended to make you to think you have to purchase every item on the list.

- It is impossible to list all the items allowed in a plant-based diet. For example, because fruits and vegetables of all kinds are allowed, there are just too many to list. Additionally, so are easier to find in some areas of the world than others so these two types of foods will vary from person to person, and country to country.

- Use the following list to help you become familiar with the items eaten and used in recipes.

- As you learn about the items used in recipes you want to make and foods you want to eat, purchase a few items at a time that will only be used occasionally. This will allow you to slowly and methodically stock your pantry with new herbs, spices, nuts, and grains.

- Try to purchase fresh produce locally whenever possible and when in season. Otherwise, consider frozen next.

- Buy organic items whenever you can afford to.

- If you are able to buy items in bulk, consider repackaging them so excess can be stored or frozen.

If you would like to have the following grocery list as a PDF so you can download it and print it out, go to http://UnitedPublishingHouse.com/wp-content/uploads/2013/07/Plant-Based-Grocery-List.pdf - and get yourself a copy.

Plant Based Grocery List

Vegetables (Fresh/organic if possible; frozen next; canned last resort)

- [ ] Asparagus
- [ ] Avocado
- [ ] Beets
- [ ] Bell peppers (sweet)
- [ ] Broccoli
- [ ] Brussels sprouts
- [ ] Cabbage
- [ ] Carrots
- [ ] Cauliflower
- [ ] Celery
- [ ] Corn
- [ ] Cucumbers
- [ ] Eggplant
- [ ] Garlic
- [ ] Ginger
- [ ] Green beans
- [ ] Kale
- [ ] Lemons
- [ ] Lettuces (all kinds)
- [ ] Limes
- [ ] Mushrooms
- [ ] Mustard greens
- [ ] Okra
- [ ] Onions
- [ ] Potatoes (all kinds)
- [ ] Pumpkin
- [ ] Radishes
- [ ] Shallots
- [ ] Snowpeas
- [ ] Spinach
- [ ] Sprouts (Broccoli, Alfalfa, etc.)
- [ ] Squash (acorn, butternut, spaghetti, etc.)
- [ ] Tomatoes
- [ ] Turnip greens
- [ ] Zucchini

Fruits (Fresh/organic if possible; frozen next; canned last resort)

- [ ] Apples
- [ ] Bananas
- [ ] Berries—all kinds
- [ ] Cherries
- [ ] Cranberries
- [ ] Dates
- [ ] Figs
- [ ] Grapefruit
- [ ] Grapes
- [ ] Kiwis
- [ ] Lemons
- [ ] Limes
- [ ] Mangoes
- [ ] Melons (watermelon, cantaloupe, etc.)
- [ ] Nectarines
- [ ] Oranges
- [ ] Papaya
- [ ] Peaches
- [ ] Pears
- [ ] Pineapple
- [ ] Plums
- [ ] Tangerines

Dried Foods

- [ ] Apples
- [ ] Apricots
- [ ] Cranberries
- [ ] Dates
- [ ] Figs
- [ ] Peaches
- [ ] Pears
- [ ] Raisins
- [ ] Tomatoes

Grains/Flours/Rices/Beans

- [ ] All purpose flour
- [ ] Brown lentils
- [ ] Brown rice
- [ ] Chick-pea flour
- [ ] Cornmeal
- [ ] Farro
- [ ] Plain oatmeal (without all the additives)
- [ ] Popcorn
- [ ] Quinoa
- [ ] Red lentils
- [ ] Rolled oats
- [ ] Rye
- [ ] Spelt
- [ ] Split peas
- [ ] Wheat germ
- [ ] 100% whole wheat bread
- [ ] Whole wheat couscous
- [ ] Whole wheat flour
- [ ] Whole wheat pasta
- [ ] Whole wheat tortillas

Dairy (if you want to find alternatives)

- [ ] Butter (substitutes like Earth Balance)
- [ ] Cheeses (substitutes like Daiya, Tofutti and Nutty Cow)
- [ ] Margarine
- [ ] Milk (almond, coconut, rice, soy)

Plant Based Grocery List

- ☐ Tofutti sour cream/cheeses
- ☐ Yogurt – coconut, soy or almond

Eggs

- ☐ Ener-G Egg Replacer and The Vegg for recipes

Protein (and meat substitutes)

- ☐ Amy's frozen products
- ☐ Beans (black, kidney, navy, etc.)
- ☐ Gardein products
- ☐ Lentils
- ☐ Protein powder (plant-based)
- ☐ Seitan
- ☐ Tempeh
- ☐ Tofu
- ☐ Tofurkey (faux meats like turkey and sausage)

Nuts/Seeds/Butters

- ☐ Almonds
- ☐ Almond butter
- ☐ Brazil nuts
- ☐ Cashews
- ☐ Cashew butter
- ☐ Chestnuts
- ☐ Flax seeds (whole and ground)
- ☐ Hazelnuts
- ☐ Macadamia nuts
- ☐ Macadamia nut butter
- ☐ Peanuts
- ☐ Peanut butter
- ☐ Pecans

- ☐ Pecan butter
- ☐ Pine nuts
- ☐ Pistachio
- ☐ Pumpkin seeds
- ☐ Sesame seeds
- ☐ Soy nuts
- ☐ Sunflower seeds
- ☐ Tahini
- ☐ Walnuts
- ☐ Walnut butter

Canned Products

- ☐ Adzuki beans
- ☐ Artichoke hearts
- ☐ Black beans
- ☐ Black eyed peas
- ☐ Cannellini beans
- ☐ Chickpeas
- ☐ Coconut milk
- ☐ Corn
- ☐ Garbanzo beans
- ☐ Pinto beans
- ☐ Pumpkin (100% pureed)
- ☐ Tomatoes (diced, paste, stewed, etc.)

Oils and Vinegars

- ☐ Almond oil
- ☐ Apple cider vinegar
- ☐ Balsamic vinegar
- ☐ Canola oil
- ☐ Coconut oil
- ☐ Corn oil
- ☐ Cottonseed oil
- ☐ Olive oil
- ☐ Peanut oil

- ☐ Rice vinegar
- ☐ Safflower oil
- ☐ Sesame oil
- ☐ Soybean oil
- ☐ Sunflower oil
- ☐ Walnut oil
- ☐ Wine vinegars (red wine, white, sherry, etc.)

Sugar/Condiments/Sauces

- ☐ Agave nectar
- ☐ Arrowroot/corn starch
- ☐ Baking soda
- ☐ Baking powder
- ☐ Barbecue sauce
- ☐ Capers
- ☐ Confectioner's sugar
- ☐ Dijon mustard
- ☐ Earth Balance products
- ☐ Ketchup
- ☐ Maple syrup
- ☐ Mayonnaise (canola or Veganaise)
- ☐ Mirin
- ☐ Miso paste
- ☐ Molasses
- ☐ Mustard
- ☐ Olives
- ☐ Pickles
- ☐ Sea salt
- ☐ Soy sauce or tamari
- ☐ Spaghetti sauce (meatless)
- ☐ Stevia
- ☐ Sucanat
- ☐ Sugars (brown, white, etc.)
- ☐ Teriyaki

Plant Based Grocery List

- ☐ Truvia
- ☐ Vanilla extract
- ☐ Vegan Worcestershire sauce

Spices/Herbs

- ☐ Bay leaves
- ☐ Cardamom
- ☐ Cayenne powder
- ☐ Celery seed
- ☐ Chili powder
- ☐ Cinnamon (ground/sticks)
- ☐ Cloves (ground/whole)
- ☐ Coriander
- ☐ Cumin (ground/seeds)
- ☐ Curry powder
- ☐ Dill (weed/seeds)
- ☐ Fennel seeds
- ☐ Garam masala
- ☐ Ginger (ground)
- ☐ Marjoram
- ☐ Mustard (dry/seeds)
- ☐ Nutmeg
- ☐ Oregano
- ☐ Paprika
- ☐ Parsley
- ☐ Peppercorns
- ☐ Rosemary
- ☐ Sage
- ☐ Tarragon
- ☐ Thyme
- ☐ Turmeric

Frozen Foods

- ☐ Bagels
- ☐ Fruits (all kinds without additives)
- ☐ Meat Substitutes
- ☐ Pizza (vegan/vegetarian)
- ☐ Vegetables (all kinds without additives)

Miscellaneous Items

- ☐ Bacon bits (meatless)
- ☐ Bouillon (vegetable)
- ☐ Cacao powder/cocoa powder
- ☐ Carob (chips and powder)
- ☐ Chocolate chips (dark)
- ☐ Coconut (flakes, shredded)
- ☐ Coffee (organic if possible)
- ☐ Jellies, jams and preserves
- ☐ Nutritional yeast
- ☐ Shortening
- ☐ Teas
- ☐ Yeast

In Summary

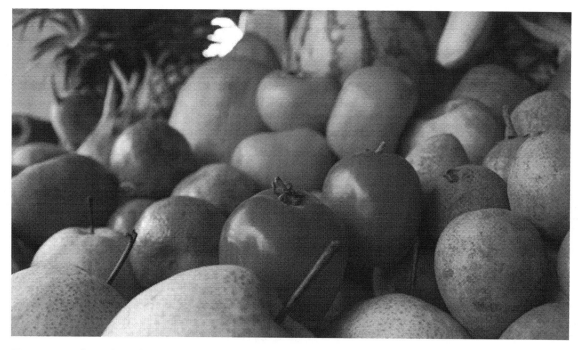

To summarize, the plant based recipes from this series will help broaden your food choices and help you find some new favorites as you begin, or continue, your journey in this style of eating.

As you read through the recipes, remember they are written for all types of plant-based eaters which means you may want to make your own substitutions if you don't eat dairy and eggs. With so many options available, this should not prove difficult even if you are a beginner. If a recipe appears to be "too much trouble," then just skip it, find another one that looks easier and make that. Come back to the recipe you skipped at a later date when your confidence has increased.

And while you are looking through the recipes in this cookbook, consider enjoying breakfast and lunch recipes for dinner or save your dinner leftovers and enjoy them for lunch the next day. No matter how you do it, you will enjoy many of the recipes included in this cookbook.

As you make adjustments in your diet, remember you are making positive changes so have a good attitude, incorporate a sense of adventure, and have fun!

Welcome to plant-based eating!

List of Pantry Ingredients

Here is a list of ingredients you will want to have in your pantry to make many of the recipes included in this collection.

Beginning on page 231, there is an index containing all the main ingredients used in this cookbook. Simply find the ingredient you want to use, and the page number will be listed beside the title of the recipes using that particular ingredient.

- allspice
- apple cider vinegar
- arrowroot powder
- baking powder
- baking soda
- balsamic vinegar
- basil
- bay leaves
- brown sugar
- cayenne pepper
- celery seed
- chili powder
- chipotle pepper
- chives (dried)
- cinnamon (ground)
- cloves (ground)
- cocoa powder
- coconut oil
- coriander
- cornstarch
- cream of tartar
- creole seasoning
- cumin (ground)
- curry powder
- dill weed (dried)
- dry mustard
- egg replacer (Ener-G Egg Replacer® is a good one)
- flours (all purpose, pastry, potato, tapioca, etc.)
- garlic cloves
- garlic powder
- ginger (ground)
- honey
- Italian seasoning mix
- jerk seasoning
- lemon juice
- marjoram
- Mexican seasoning

- minced onion
- nutmeg (ground)
- olive oil
- onion powder
- onions
- oregano (dried)
- paprika
- parsley (dried)
- pepper
- powdered sugar (confectioners' sugar)
- pure maple syrup
- pure vanilla extract
- red pepper flakes
- red wine vinegar
- rosemary
- sage
- salt
- soy sauce
- sugar
- thyme
- turmeric
- white vinegar

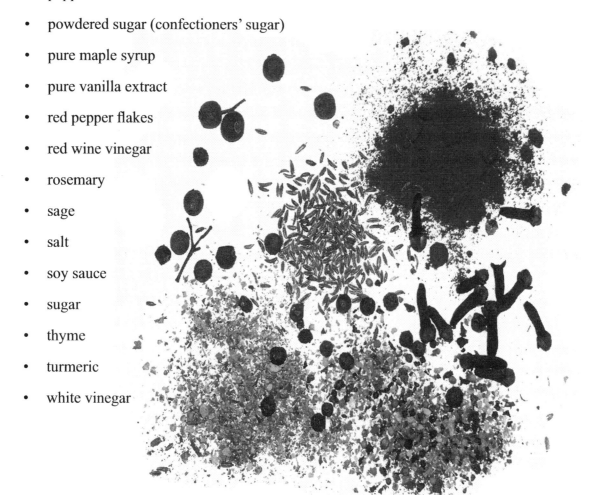

Breakfast Recipes

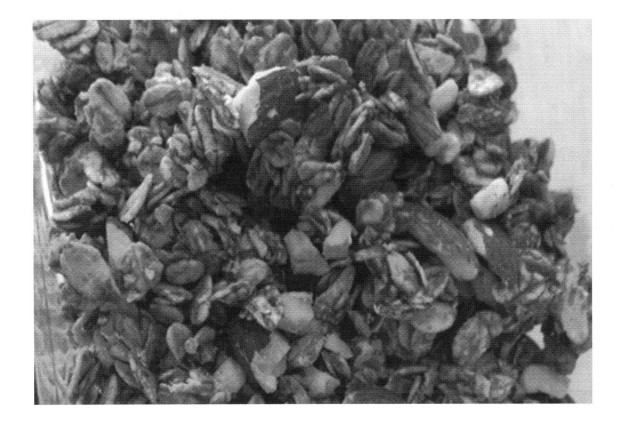

There are so many different kinds of foods you can enjoy for breakfast when eating a plant-based diet. From smoothies, to parfaits, to pancakes and waffles, there are many foods to be enjoyed. If you thought you were going to have to eat a lot of cereals to make the transition, you are in for a delightful adventure. Enjoy experimenting and creating new recipes along the way.

Cocoa Waffles

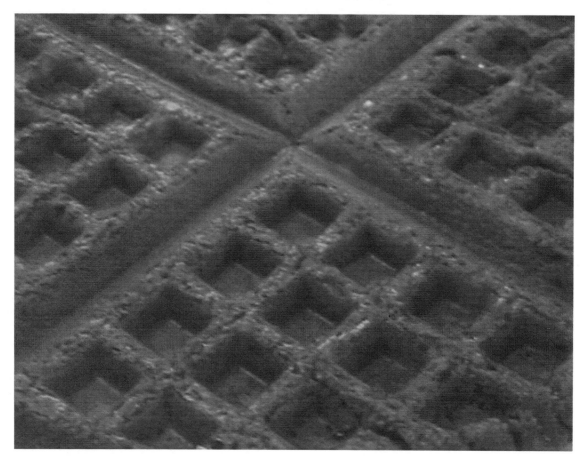

Ingredients:

- 1 cup flour

- ¾ cup sugar

- ½ cup cocoa powder

- ½ teaspoon baking powder

- ½ teaspoon baking soda

- ¼ teaspoon salt

- 2 eggs (use egg replacer here)

- 1 cup vegan buttermilk

- ¼ cup coconut oil, melted
- 1 teaspoon pure vanilla extract

Directions:

1. Preheat your waffle iron to the desired setting

2. In a medium bowl, combine the flour, sugar, cocoa, baking powder, soda, and salt

3. In a separate bowl, combine the eggs, buttermilk, melted coconut oil, and vanilla

4. Gently blend the wet ingredients in with the dry ones until the batter is a uniform consistency

5. Pour desired amount of batter onto the waffle iron and cook until browned

6. Top with your favorite topping/sweetener

Makes 4 servings

How to Make Vegan Buttermilk (makes 1 cup)

- 1 tablespoon vinegar (white or apple cider) OR lemon or lime juice
- 1 cup nut, rice or soy milk

1. Measure out 1 tablespoon of vinegar or juice and place in a measuring cup

2. Pour the milk into the measuring cup up to the 1-cup line

3. Allow to sit for 10 minutes

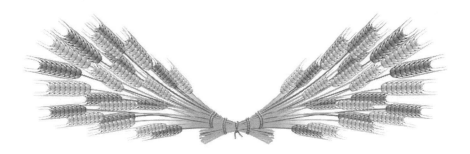

Fried Tortilla Casserole

This recipe is one my family and I often enjoy for lunch on the weekends or for a delicious dinner entrée. Make it and see what your family thinks.

Ingredients:

- 2 - 3 tablespoons coconut oil

- 6 small tortillas

- 1 large onion, chopped

- 1 garlic clove, minced

- 2 cups crumbled meat substitute

- 3 large tomatoes, chopped

- 4 ounce can green chili peppers, chopped

- ¼ teaspoon salt

- 1 cup vegan shredded cheese (your choice)

Directions:

1. Preheat your oven to broil

2. Lightly grease a rectangular baking dish that will accommodate the 6 tortillas in the bottom of it

3. In a large skillet, heat up the oil

4. Using tongs, place one tortilla at a time in the hot oil for 10 seconds, then flip and fry for another 10 seconds

5. Place each one in the bottom of your baking dish as you fry them

6. Once your tortillas are fried, melt a little bit more oil if necessary

7. Put the chopped onion, garlic and meat in the pan and sauté until tender

8. Now stir in the chopped tomatoes, green chilies, and salt

9. Cook on low for about 10 minutes

10. Place this mixture over the top of the tortillas in your baking dish

11. Now sprinkle the cheese over the top and place under your broiler until the cheese melts like you like it

Makes 6 to 8 servings

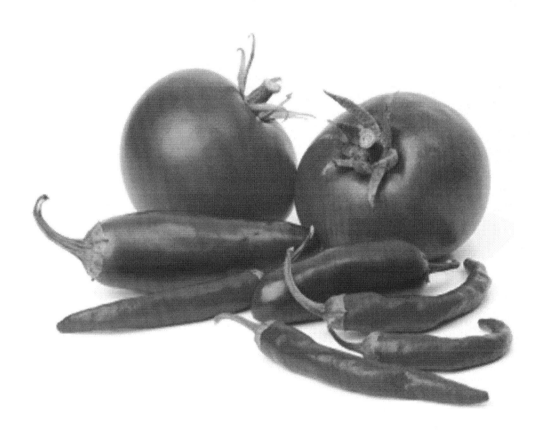

Sunrise Muffins

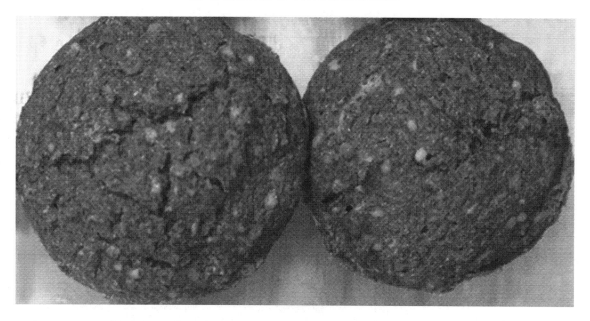

This is a delicious way to get some fruit and veggies into your breakfast. These are also great to serve with a main meal, too.

Ingredients:

- 2 cups flour

- 1 cup sugar

- 1 tablespoon ground cinnamon

- 2 teaspoons baking powder

- ½ teaspoon baking soda

- ½ teaspoon salt

- 2 cups grated carrots

- 1 apple–peeled, cored, and chopped

- 1 cup raisins

- 2 eggs (an egg replacer works fine here)

- ½ cup apple butter

- ¼ cup olive oil

- 1 tablespoon vanilla extract

- 2 tablespoons chopped walnuts

- 2 tablespoons toasted wheat germ

Directions:

1. Preheat your oven to 375 degrees F

2. Lightly grease 18 muffin cups

3. In a large bowl, combine the flour, sugar, cinnamon, baking powder, baking soda, and salt and mix well

4. Stir in the grated carrots, chopped apples, and raisins

5. In a smaller bowl, whisk together the egg replacements, apple butter, oil, and vanilla

6. Add the egg mixture to your dry ingredients and gently mix until moistened throughout

7. Spoon equal amounts of batter into each muffin cup

8. Top with walnuts and wheat germ

9. Bake in your preheated oven for 15–20 minutes or until the centers are clean with the toothpick test

10. Remove from the muffin cups when cooked and allow to cool on a cooling rack

Makes 18 muffins

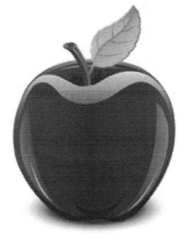

Nutty Oatmeal

The addition of nut butters to your oatmeal in the morning makes for a delightful and nutty way to clear the morning fogginess from your head and palate!

Ingredients:

- 1 cup water

- ½ cup quick cooking oats

- ½ banana, mashed

- 1 tablespoon chunky nut butter of your choice

Directions:

1. Place the water in a small saucepan and bring to a boil

2. Add the oats and cook for approximately 5 to 6 minutes

3. Once the oats are cooked, add the mashed banana and nut butter to the saucepan

4. Stir together to heat ingredients thoroughly

5. Top with your favorite milk alternative if desired

Makes 1 serving

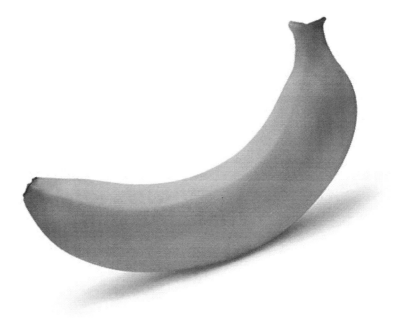

Buttery Scones

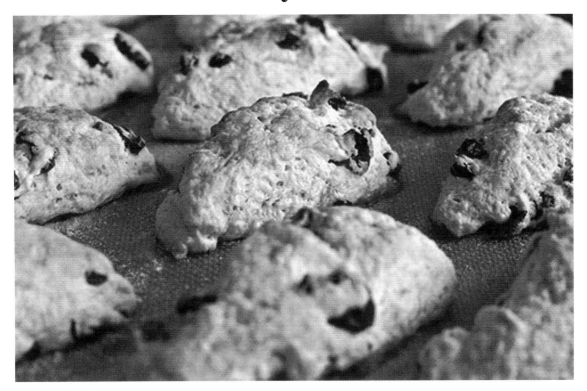

Ingredients:

- 1 cup Tofutti® sour cream

- 1 teaspoon baking soda

- 4 cups flour

- 1 cup sugar

- 2 teaspoons baking powder

- ¼ teaspoon cream of tartar

- 1 teaspoon salt

- 2 Earth Balance Buttery Sticks®

- 1 egg (use egg replacer or applesauce)

- 1 cup raisins or dried cranberries

Directions:

1. Preheat your oven to 350 degrees F

2. Lightly grease a large baking sheet

3. In a small bowl, blend the sour cream and baking soda

4. Set aside for later

5. In a large bowl, combine the flour, sugar, baking powder, cream of tartar, and salt

6. Cut in the butter until mixed throughout the flour

7. Add the egg to the flour and mix in

8. Take your sour cream mixture and mix until moistened

9. Add in the raisins or cranberries

10. Remove the dough from your bowl and place it on a lightly oiled surface

11. Knead briefly

12. Roll the dough out into a rounded shape until it is ¾ inch thick

13. Cut the dough into 12 even wedges

14. Place them onto your baking sheet approximately 2 inches apart from each other

15. Bake in your preheated oven for approximately 15 minutes

16. Scones are done when they are golden brown

Makes 12 scones

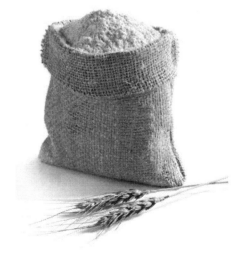

Apple Omelet

If you are a plant eater who does not eat eggs, you may want to skip this recipe. Otherwise, I highly recommend this one if you do enjoy eggs.

Ingredients:

Sauce

- ¼ cup packed brown sugar

- 1 tablespoon cornstarch

- 2/3 cup water

- 2 teaspoons lemon juice

- 3 apples–peeled, cored, and diced

- 2 tablespoons Earth Balance Buttery Sticks®

- 3 fully cooked veggie sausage links, sliced

Omelet

- 1 tablespoon Earth Balance Butter®

- 1 container tofu, firm or extra-firm – pressed and mashed

- ½ teaspoon soy sauce

- Salt to taste

- ½ cup vegan shredded cheese (your choice)

Directions:

1. Begin by combining the brown sugar and cornstarch in a saucepan over medium heat

2. Stir in the cold water and lemon juice

3. Stir constantly as the mixture thickens and bubbles

4. Now add the apples and stir gently

5. Cover the saucepan and simmer gently for 5 minutes or until the apples are tender

6. Once the apples are tender, add the butter and veggie sausage

7. Stir until the butter melts and the sausage gets hot

8. Cover to keep warm while you prepare the omelet

9. In a separate frying pan, heat up the butter

10. Now put in the mashed tofu and soy sauce

11. Sauté for 6 to 7 minutes, stirring frequently so it doesn't burn

12. Pour your apple mixture on top of the tofu

13. Now sprinkle the cheese over the apples

14. Continue to heat gently until the cheese melts

Makes 4 servings

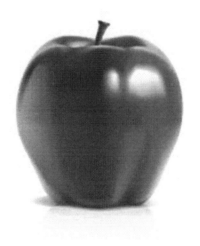

Pumpkin Bread

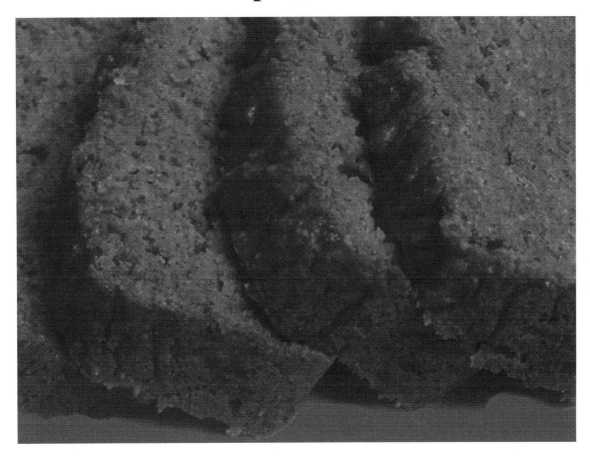

Pumpkin bread can be made any time of the year when you have access to canned pumpkin. This recipe is so delicious, you will find yourself wanting to make it on a regular basis.

Ingredients:

- 1 (15 ounce) can 100% pumpkin puree

- 4 eggs (use egg replacement)

- 1 cup coconut oil, melted

- 2/3 cup water

- 2 cups sugar

- 3½ cups flour

- 2 teaspoons baking soda

- 1½ teaspoons salt

- 1 teaspoon ground cinnamon

- 1 teaspoon ground nutmeg

- ½ teaspoon ground cloves

- ¼ teaspoon ground ginger

Directions:

1. Preheat your oven to 350 degrees F

2. Lightly grease and flour 3 regular-sized loaf pans

3. In a large bowl, mix together the pumpkin, egg replacer, oil, water and sugar until combined thoroughly

4. In a separate bowl, whisk together the flour, soda, salt, cinnamon, nutmeg, cloves and ginger

5. Gently stir the dry ingredients into the pumpkin mixture until just blended

6. Pour into the prepared pans, dividing the batter evenly

7. Bake for 45–50 minutes in your oven

8. Loaves are done

Makes 3 loaves

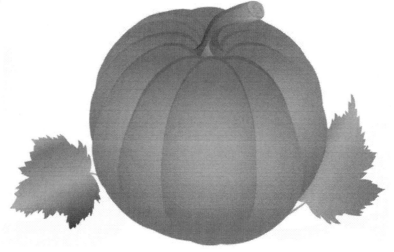

Chocolate Burrito

Chocolate for breakfast? Sure! With the addition of some granola cereal, this is truly a treat for breakfast!

Ingredients:

- ½ tablespoon coconut oil
- 1 large flour tortilla
- ¼ ounce vegan unsweetened chocolate, chopped into small pieces
- ½ tablespoon powdered sugar
- ½ cup favorite granola-type cereal
- ¼ cup nuts, chopped
- ½ tablespoon pure maple syrup

Directions:

1. On a flat griddle or frying pan, melt the coconut oil
2. Once heated, place the tortilla on the griddle and let the oil soak in
3. Place the chocolate on top of the tortilla. It should melt if the tortilla is heated through
4. Now sprinkle on the powdered sugar and gently stir the two ingredients together on top of the tortilla
5. Sprinkle the cereal and chopped nuts into the center of the tortilla along the centerfold
6. Fold the ends of the tortilla inward toward the middle so it is divided into thirds
7. Allow the tortilla to continue to heat for another minute
8. Remove from the heat and put the tortilla on a plate
9. Lightly drizzle the maple syrup over the tortilla and enjoy

Makes 1 serving

Cheese Grits

Ingredients:

- 3 cups water

- ½ teaspoon salt

- 1 cup hominy grits

- ¼ teaspoon pepper

- 1 tablespoon Earth Balance Buttery Sticks®

- ½ cup vegan shredded cheese

- 4 strips vegan bacon (cooked and crumbled)

Directions:

1. In a medium saucepan, bring the water and salt to a boil

2. Quickly add in the grits and stir continually until the mixture comes to a boil

3. Turn the heat down to low

4. Cook for an additional 15 minutes, stirring occasionally

5. Once the grits are cooked, add the pepper, butter, and cheese

6. Mix thoroughly, allowing the butter and cheese to melt

7. Sprinkle the bacon crumbles on top

Makes 3 to 4 servings

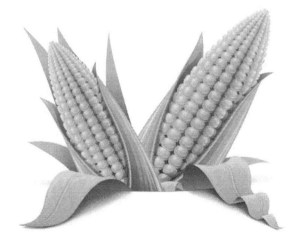

Potato Pancakes

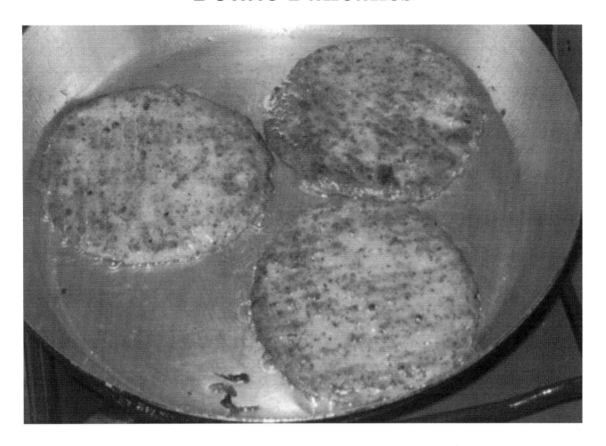

Ingredients:

- 5 large red skinned potatoes

- 1 onion

- ½ cup chickpea flour (can be made by grinding chickpeas in a food processor, coffee grinder or blender)

- 1 tablespoon water (optional)

- Coconut oil for frying

Directions:

1. Begin by grating the potatoes using a food processor or hand grater until you have shredded 3 full cups worth

2. Finely chop the onion or you can also process them in the food processor

3. Combine both the potatoes and onions together into a medium bowl

4. Taking about one cup full of the potato/onion mixture, compress between your hands and squeeze out excess moisture

5. After mixture has been squeezed, mix the potato mixture in the bowl with the chick-pea flour until moistened

6. Using a large melon ball scoop or a large tablespoon, scoop out a golf-sized amount of potato mixture

7. Squeeze and press into a ball. If it won't hold its shape, you need a little moisture replaced so add small amounts of water until mixture is moist enough

8. Continue forming balls until the mixture is used up

9. Take a frying pan and fill with oil so the oil is just over ¼ inch deep

10. Heat over medium-high heat

11. Take each golf-ball shaped potato and flatten into a patty with your hands and gently place into the hot oil

12. Cook the patties on each side for 5 minutes until they are golden brown

13. Can be enjoyed plain or with a favorite topping

Makes 4 to 5 servings

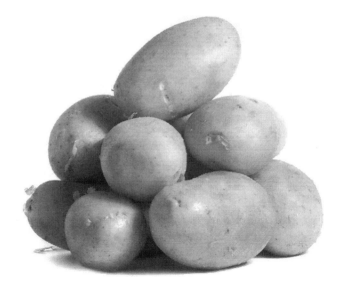

Delicious Breakfast Burritos

Ingredients:

- 2 tablespoons Earth Balance Buttery Sticks®

- 2 red potatoes, diced

- Salt & pepper to taste

- 1 onion, chopped

- 2 garlic cloves, minced

- 1 block extra-firm tofu

- 2 tablespoon turmeric

- 2 tablespoon cumin

- 1 tablespoon coriander

- 2 tablespoon soy sauce

- 1 tablespoon coconut oil

- 4 large flour tortillas

Directions:

1. In a medium frying pan, melt the butter

2. Add the potatoes, salt, and pepper

3. Fry until the potatoes are golden brown and thoroughly cooked

4. Now add the onion and garlic and cook for 2 to 3 more minutes

5. Squeeze the excess water from the tofu and crumble it into your frying pan

6. Add the turmeric, cumin, and coriander

7. Stir for 2 to 3 minutes

8. In the center of the pan, make a small indentation and pour the soy sauce into it and heat thoroughly

9. In a separate frying pan, add a small amount of oil

10. Heat each tortilla for 30 seconds on each side

11. Place on a paper towel to drain

12. Place each tortilla on a plate and add the tofu mixture

13. Roll up like a burrito and enjoy

Makes 4 servings

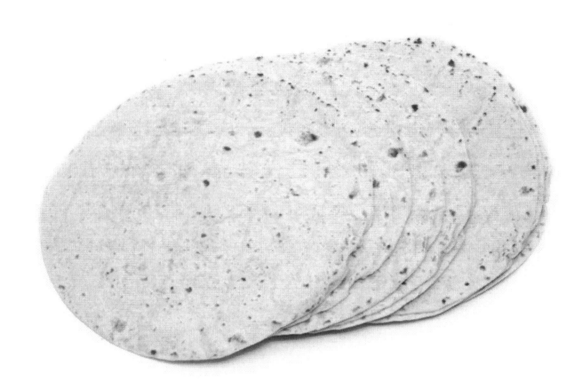

Red Pita Pockets

Ingredients:

- 2 tablespoons coconut oil

- 2 cups red potatoes, cooked and diced

- 1 small onion, chopped

- 1 red bell pepper, chopped

- 1 block extra-firm tofu

- Salt and pepper to taste

- 4 pita bread, cut in half

Directions:

1. In a medium frying pan, melt the oil

2. Now add the potatoes, onion, and bell pepper

3. Cook until the vegetables are soft

4. Squeeze the excess water from the tofu and crumble it into your frying pan with the vegetables

5. Season with salt and pepper

6. Continue cooking while chopping the tofu into little pieces as it cooks

7. Warm the pita bread briefly in your microwave

8. Once your tofu/vegetable mixture is done, stuff each half of the pita with the mixture

Makes 8 pockets

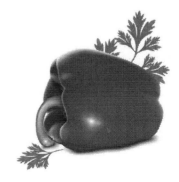

Banana Bread

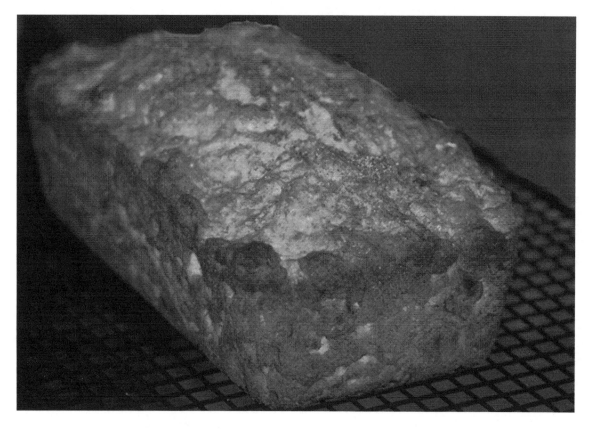

How nice that you can still enjoy a delicious, warm piece of banana bread--even on a plant-based diet. Enjoy this one any time of day. It is also a great complement to any dinner recipe, too.

Ingredients:

- 2 eggs (use egg replacer here)

- 1/3 cup vegan buttermilk

- ½ cup coconut oil

- 1 cup mashed bananas

- 1 cup sugar

- 1¾ cups flour

- 1 teaspoon baking soda
- ½ teaspoon salt
- ½ cup chopped pecans

Directions:

1. Preheat your oven to 325 degrees F

2. Spray a 9 x 5 inch loaf pan with non-stick spray coating

3. In a medium bowl, use a hand mixer and blend the eggs, buttermilk, oil, and bananas together

4. In a separate bowl, mix the sugar, flour, baking soda, and salt until well blended

5. Add the flour mixture to the banana mixture and blend on low until thoroughly mixed

6. Briefly mix in the pecans

7. Pour the batter into your prepared loaf pan and bake for 70 to 80 minutes or until a cake tester comes out clean when inserted in the middle

8. Remove from the oven when done

9. Gently dump the loaf out onto a cooling rack and allow to cool completely before cutting

Makes 1 loaf

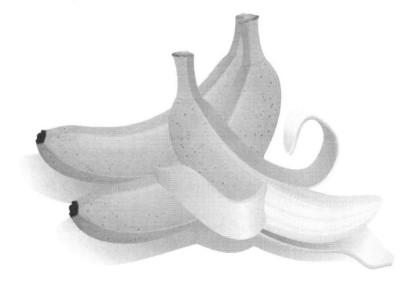

Coco-Nutty Toast

Ingredients:

- 2 tablespoons powdered sugar

- 2 teaspoons ground cinnamon

- 2 tablespoons shredded coconut

- 2 slices of whole grain bread

- 2 tablespoons Earth Balance Buttery Sticks®

Directions:

1. Place your oven on broil

2. Combine the sugar, cinnamon, and coconut in a shallow dish

3. Lightly toasting your bread in a toaster or under the broiler once it is hot. (You want to get it hot enough to melt the butter)

4. Once it is toasted, spread butter on each side of the bread

5. Cut into strips

6. Roll the strips into the coconut mixture, making sure some sticks to the sides of the strips

7. Place the strips on a pan and put under the broiler

8. Turn the strips as each side browns to your liking

9. Top with maple syrup or fruit preserves

Makes 1 to 2 servings

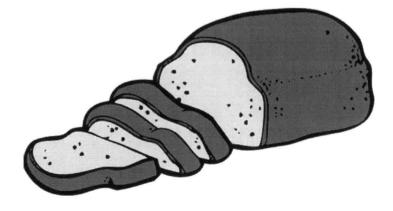

Homemade Granola

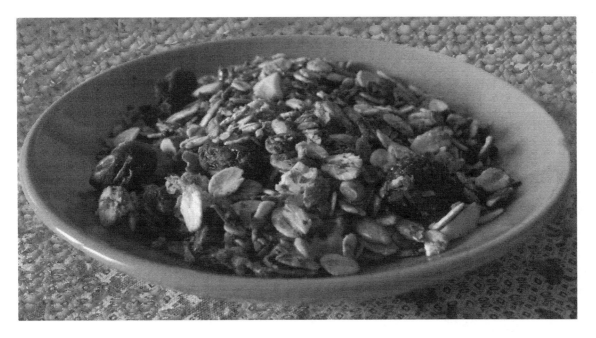

This recipe is not only delicious for a breakfast cereal, but it also makes a great snack you can munch on during the day.

Ingredients:

- 8 cups rolled oats

- 1½ cups oat bran

- 1½ cups wheat germ

- 1 cup finely chopped almonds

- 1 cup finely chopped pecans

- 1 cup finely chopped walnuts

- 1 cup sunflower seeds

- 2 cups raisins or sweetened dried cranberries

- ½ cup brown sugar

- 1½ teaspoons salt

- ¾ cup honey (raw if you can find it)

- 1 tablespoon pure vanilla extract

- 1 cup coconut or olive oil

- 1 tablespoon ground cinnamon

Directions:

1. Preheat your oven to 325 degrees F

2. Take two large cookie sheets or baking sheets that have a lip around the edges and line them with parchment paper or aluminum foil

3. In a large bowl, combine the oats, oat bran, wheat germ, almonds, pecans, walnuts, sunflower seeds, raisins/cranberries and mix thoroughly

4. In a medium saucepan, combine the brown sugar, salt, honey, vanilla, oil, and cinnamon and cook over medium-high heat

5. Bring to a boil

6. Now pour the hot liquid over the dry ingredients and stir until mixed thoroughly

7. Pour the mixture out onto the baking sheets and spread out evenly

8. Place the sheets into your preheated oven and bake for approximately 20–25 minutes.

9. Turn the granola over gently with a big spoon until the liquid has been absorbed into the grains and the granola is dry and crispy

10. Remove from the oven

11. Allow the granola to cool, then store in airtight containers

Makes 15 to 16 cups granola

Salsa Breakfast Burritos

Ingredients:

- 1 (15 ounce) can black beans, drained

- 2 tablespoons olive or coconut oil

- 1 pound veggie sausage

- 1 (10 count) package 10-inch flour tortillas

- 1½ cups vegan shredded cheese

- 1 (16 ounce) jar of your favorite salsa

Directions:

1. Empty the black beans into a microwave-safe dish

2. Process until they are heated through

3. Place the oil into a large skillet

4. Once the oil is hot, add the sausage and cook thoroughly

5. Remove the tortillas from the package

6. For each tortilla, place a desired amount of black beans on each one, followed by sausage, shredded cheese, and a spoonful of salsa

7. Roll each tortilla up like a burrito

Makes 10 burritos

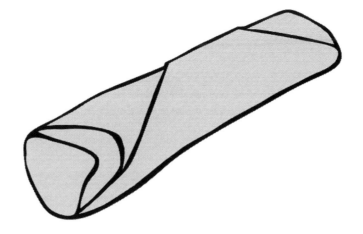

Top of the Morning Pancakes

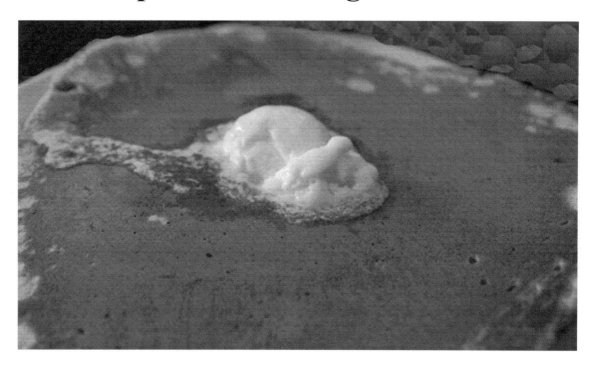

Ingredients

- 2 cups flour
- ½ teaspoon baking soda
- 1 tablespoon sugar
- 1 teaspoon baking powder
- 1 2/3 cups soy, rice or nut milk
- 2 tablespoons coconut oil

Directions

1. In a medium-sized bowl, mix together the flour, baking soda, sugar, and baking powder

2. Add to the dry ingredients the milk and oil

3. On a griddle, melt 1 - 2 additional tablespoons of coconut oil

4. When hot, pour 1/8 to 1/4 cup of batter onto the griddle and spread out the batter with the back of a spoon if needed

5. When the batter begins to bubble and look dry along the edges, flip over and brown on the other side

6. Top with delicious maple syrup or your favorite fruit topping

Makes 8 to 12 pancakes

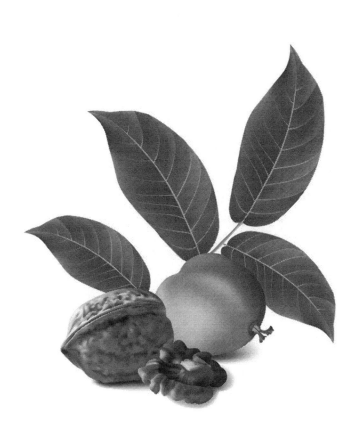

Breakfast in a Pan

If you are okay using eggs, this is a delicious omelet. However, you can definitely use tofu if you prefer

Ingredients:

- 1–2 tablespoons Earth Balance Butter®

- 1 (14 ounce) package extra-firm tofu (drained)

- 2 tablespoons nut, rice, or soy milk

- 1 onion, chopped

- 6 strips veggie bacon, cut into slices

- Salt and pepper to taste

- 1 garlic clove, minced

- 1 cup vegan shredded cheese

Directions:

1. In a large skillet, melt the butter over medium heat

2. In a large bowl, crumble the tofu and mix with milk

3. Place the onion, bacon, salt, pepper and garlic into the skillet and cook until bacon and onions are done

4. Pour the tofu over the contents in your skillet

5. Continue to sauté with the rest of the mixture

6. Now add the cheese and stir until melted in with the rest of your mixture

7. Serve when heated through

Makes 3 to 4 servings

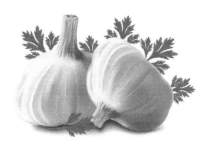

Orange You Glad Muffins

Ingredients

- 1 cup whole wheat flour
- 1 cup oat bran
- 1 teaspoon baking powder
- 1 teaspoon baking soda
- 1 teaspoon allspice
- ½ teaspoon ground cinnamon
- 1 tablespoon cornstarch
- 2/3 cup grated carrots
- 1 cup water
- ¼ cup coconut oil
- 1/3 cup pure maple syrup

Directions

1. Preheat your oven to 375 degrees F
2. Lightly spray a 12-cup muffin tin with non-stick coating spray
3. In a large bowl, combine the flour, oat bran, baking powder, baking soda, allspice, cinnamon, and cornstarch
4. Now add in the grated carrots and mix until the carrots are coated with flour
5. In a separate bowl, mix the water, oil and syrup together
6. Add the wet ingredients to the dry ones
7. Mix thoroughly
8. Evenly divide the batter among the muffin tins
9. Place in your preheated oven and bake for approximately 25 to 30 minutes
10. Allow to cool in the pan for 5 to 10 minutes, then dump out onto a cooling rack

Makes 12 muffins

Yummy French Toast

Here is a recipe you will want to make the night before if you are going to enjoy it for breakfast. However, consider putting the ingredients together in the morning before you leave the house; then bake it for dinner when you get home. It is terrific at any meal!

Ingredients:

1 loaf French bread, sliced

1½ cups silken tofu

1½ cups nut, rice, or soy milk

1 tablespoon pure vanilla extract

6 apples–peeled, cored and sliced

1½ teaspoons ground cinnamon

½ teaspoon ground nutmeg

2 tablespoons sugar

Sauce

- ¼ cup flour

- 1 stick of Earth Balance Butter®, melted

- ¼ cup brown sugar

- ½ cup nut, rice, or soy milk

- 2 teaspoons pure vanilla extract

Directions:

1. Take your loaf of bread and cut it into 1½-inch thick slices

2. Spray the bottom of a 9 x 13 inch baking dish with non-stick cooking spray

3. In the bottom of the baking dish, place the bread slices snugly beside each other

4. In a blender, combine the tofu, milk, and vanilla

5. Once thoroughly blended, pour this mixture over the bread slices

6. Arrange the apple slices on top of the bread slices

7. Combine the cinnamon, nutmeg, and sugar and mix together

8. Now sprinkle this mixture over the apples

9. Cover the baking dish and refrigerate overnight

10. In the morning, preheat your oven to 350 degrees F

11. Remove the baking dish from the refrigerator and place it in your preheated oven

12. Bake for 1 hour

13. In a small saucepan over medium heat, combine the flour and butter

14. Stir in the brown sugar, milk, and vanilla

15. Cook until thick

16. Remove the baking dish from the oven when the casserole is browned

17. Pour the sugar sauce over the French toast and serve

Makes 8 to 10 servings

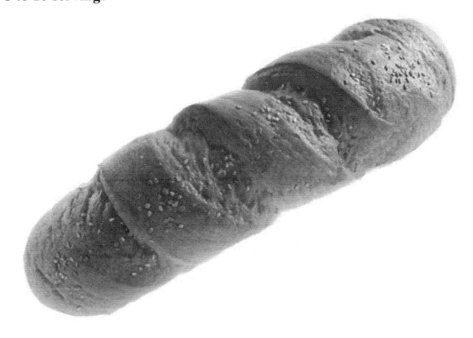

Blue Banana Smoothie

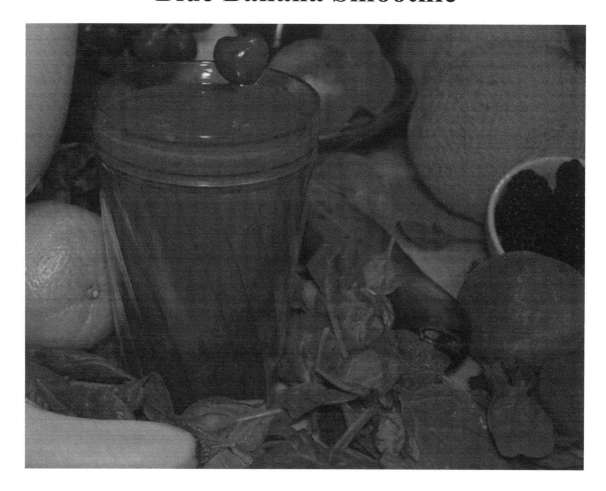

Smoothies are a delicious and nutritious way to start your day. Give this one a try. It is scrumptious!

Ingredients

- 1½ cups orange juice

- 1 cup blueberries, frozen

- 2 medium bananas, frozen

- 1 teaspoon pure vanilla extract

- 2 scoops favorite vegan protein powder

Directions

1. In a blender, pour the orange juice

2. Then add the blueberries, bananas and vanilla

3. Blend until frozen fruit is pureed. (It may be necessary to add a little more orange juice to get the fluidity you desire.)

4. Stop your blender and add in the protein powder

5. Turn on the blender again and blend only until the powder is dissolved. This will keep from making the drink foamy; however, keep blending if you like foam

Makes 2 delicious servings

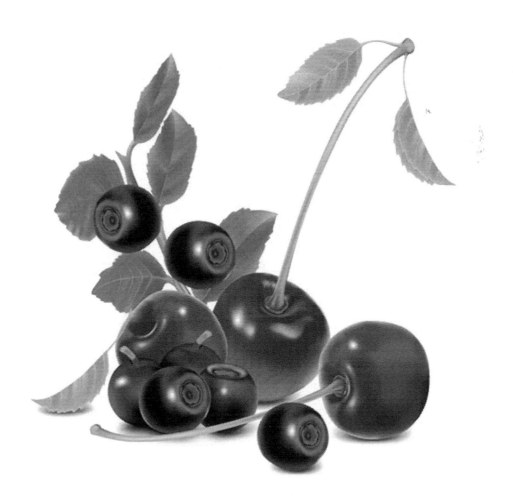

Breakfast Rice Cereal

If you find you have some leftover rice, or can make enough the night before knowing you will have this for breakfast, you can have a wonderful treat to start your day.

Ingredients

- 1 cup cooked brown rice

- 2 tablespoons shredded coconut

- 2 tablespoons chopped pecans (or your favorite nut)

- 1 tablespoon of dried cranberries or raisins

- ¼ teaspoon cinnamon

- 1 teaspoon brown sugar

- Coconut, rice, almond, or soy milk if desired

Directions

1. In a microwavable bowl, combine the rice, coconut, pecans, cranberries, cinnamon and brown sugar

2. Heat in your microwave to a temperature you like

3. Top with milk if desired

Makes 1 serving

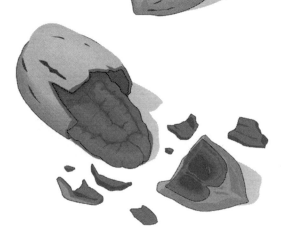

Delicious Blueberry Muffins

Ingredients

- ½ cup sugar

- 1 cup unsweetened applesauce

- 2 ripe bananas

- 1 tablespoon coconut or almond milk

- 1 teaspoon pure vanilla extract

- 2 cups whole wheat pastry flour

- 1 teaspoon baking soda

- ¼ teaspoon salt

- 1 cup blueberries, fresh or frozen - defrosted

- ½ cup nuts (walnuts or pecans)

Directions

1. Preheat your oven to 350 degrees F

2. Lightly spray a 12-cup muffin tin with non-stick cooking spray

3. In a blender, add the sugar, applesauce, bananas, milk, and vanilla and blend until thoroughly combined

4. In a medium-sized bowl, combine together the flour, baking soda, and salt

5. Add the wet ingredients from the blender to the dry ingredients and mix gently until the dry ingredients are wet

6. Now add the blueberries and nuts and stir gently again

7. Evenly divide the batter into the muffin tins

8. Place the filled muffin tins into your preheated oven

9. Bake for 20 to 25 minutes, until the center of the muffins is cooked

10. Remove the tins from the oven and let them remain in the tins for 5 to 10 minutes while they cool

11. Remove from the tins and place on a cooling rack to finish cooling

Makes 12 muffins

You could also use a regular bread loaf pan. Put the batter into a lightly-greased loaf pan, place in the oven, and bake for 45 minutes. Test the center for doneness; then cool completely before slicing.

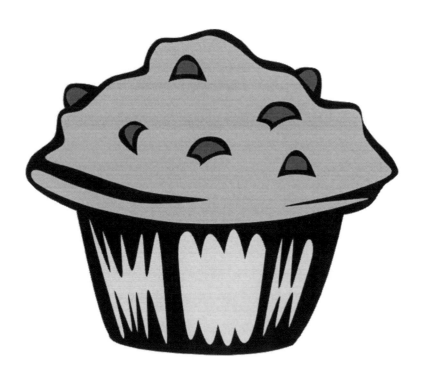

Breakfast Sweet Potato Pie

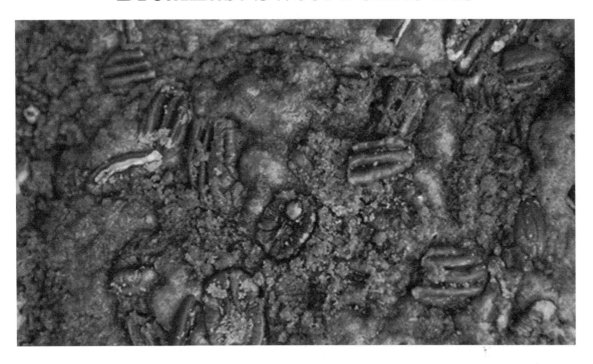

This is such a tasty recipe and one where you can use leftover sweet potatoes from last night's dinner. A delicious way to recycle.

Ingredients

- 1¾ cups coconut, almond, or soy milk

- ½ cup uncooked oats

- 1 large banana

- 1½ cups cooked sweet potatoes

- 1/8 cup pure maple syrup

- 1½ teaspoons pure vanilla extract

- 1 teaspoon ground cinnamon

- ¼ teaspoon nutmeg

- ½ teaspoon salt

Topping

- ½ cup walnuts or pecans, whole or chopped

- 2 tablespoons flour

- ¼ cup brown sugar

- 2 tablespoons Earth Balance Butter®

Directions

1. Preheat your oven to 350 degrees F

2. Using a medium pot on your stovetop, place the milk and oats

3. Bring mixture to a boil, stirring frequently

4. Lower the heat to low and cook for 6 to 7 minutes

5. Gently add the banana and sweet potato and mash them in with the oats and milk

6. Add the syrup, vanilla, cinnamon, nutmeg and salt to the pot and stir completely

7. Cook for another 5 to 6 minutes

8. Remove from heat

9. Pour the oats into an 8" x 8" baking dish that has been treated with non-stick cooking spray

10. In a medium-sized bowl, combine the nuts, flour, and brown sugar

11. Using a fork, work the butter into the mixture until it has a crumbly consistency

12. Sprinkle the brown sugar topping over the oatmeal

13. Place in your preheated oven for 20 to 25 minutes

14. Now turn your oven on BROIL and allow the topping to brown nicely. Keep a close eye on it so it does not burn

Makes 4 servings

One Omelet Coming Up

If you didn't think you would be able to enjoy another omelet when you gave up eggs, think again! This omelet has a creamy consistency and is delicious with all kinds of different fillings. You are only limited by your imagination on this one. Just make sure your pan is nice and hot before you add the batter.

Ingredients

- 2 tablespoons coconut oil

- ¼ cup sliced mushrooms

- 3 tablespoons chopped onion

- ¼ sweet bell pepper, small dices

- 1 tablespoon coconut, almond or soy milk

- ½ package (6 ounces) extra-firm silken tofu

- 1 teaspoon tahini

- 1 tablespoon nutritional yeast

- 1 tablespoon cornstarch

- 1/8 teaspoon turmeric

- 1/8 teaspoon onion powder

- ½ teaspoon salt

Directions

1. In a non-stick frying pan, melt the coconut oil

2. Add the mushrooms, onion, and pepper to the hot oil

3. Sauté the vegetables until tender

4. Remove from the heat and place in a small bowl

5. In a blender, add the milk, tofu, tahini, yeast, cornstarch, turmeric, onion powder, and salt and process until thoroughly blended

6. Place your frying pan back on the stovetop over medium heat

7. Add a little more coconut oil to the pan if needed and heat until very hot

8. Pour your batter from the blender into the middle of the frying pan and gently rotate your pan in a circular motion, causing the batter to spread out over the bottom of the pan

9. It may be necessary to smooth out your batter with a spatula or bottom of a spoon

10. Now place your sautéed vegetables in the middle of the batter and reduce the heat to medium or slightly lower

11. Cook your omelet like this for 4 to 5 minutes. You want the edges of the omelet to dry out and to cook the middle so it is not runny

12. When you think it looks done, fold one side of the omelet over the other, enclosing the filling in the middle

13. Let it remain in this position for an additional minute or two, then remove carefully from the pan

14. Your omelet is ready to be enjoyed!

Makes 1 omelet

Please note: This recipe can be doubled, but only cook one omelet's worth of batter at a time.

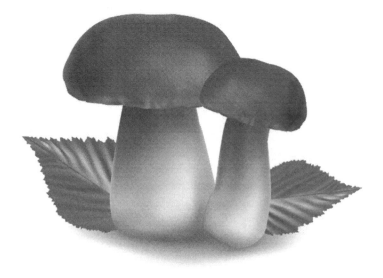

Cheesy Apple Toast

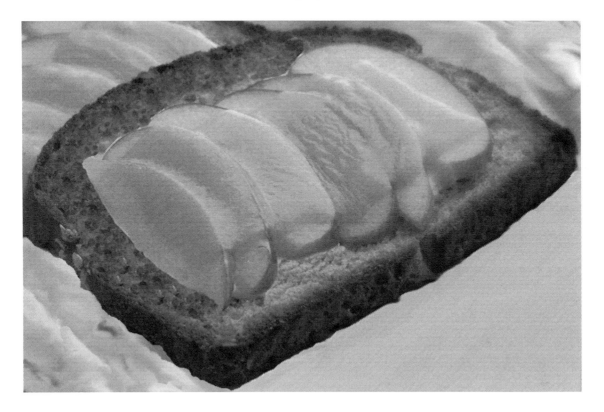

Here is a recipe that has so many possibilities for variations. To get you started, here is a delightful combination of apples with cheese to start off your morning in a delicious way. In addition, after you make this for one or two people, you could easily line the bottom of your baking sheet with pieces of toast and make like an entire casserole!

Ingredients

- 2 slices whole wheat bread, toasted

- 1 tablespoon Earth Balance Butter®

- 1 apple, thinly sliced or grated

- 2 slices vegan sliced cheese

- Sunflower seeds or other nuts (optional)

Directions

1. Preheat your oven on broil

2. Place the shelf in the middle of the oven so it is not too close to the flames

3. Take a small baking sheet and place your two pieces of toast on it

4. Spread the butter on top of the bread

5. Now place the apple on top of the butter to your liking

6. If you wish, you can sprinkle on some sunflower seeds, chopped walnuts or pecans, etc.

7. Place one slice of cheese on top of the apple for each piece of bread

8. Place the baking sheet under the broiler

9. Allow the broiler to melt the cheese until it begin to brown and bubble. Be sure to keep a close watch on it so it doesn't burn

10. Let the toast cool slightly, then eat

You could even take the two pieces of bread and make it into a sandwich!

Makes 2 pieces for one or two people

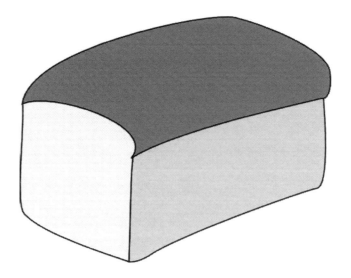

Cereal Yogurt Parfait

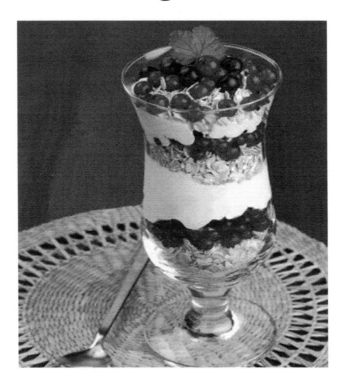

This lovely breakfast is almost like having a dessert. Filled with colorful blueberries and red currants (or cherries), the yogurt and cornflakes (or granola) make a delicious combination of flavors and textures.

Ingredients

- 1 cup corn flakes or granola
- 1 cup cherries, pitted or red currants
- 1 cup blueberries
- 2 cups flavored soy yogurt (your choice)
- ½ cup chopped nuts (optional)

Directions

1. Using two parfait glasses, place ¼ cup cornflakes (or granola) in the bottom of the glasses

2. On top of the cereal, add ¼ cup cherries and ¼ cup blueberries

3. Now put ½ cup yogurt and sprinkle nuts here if desired

4. Repeat the layering one more time

5. Eat immediately

Makes 2 servings

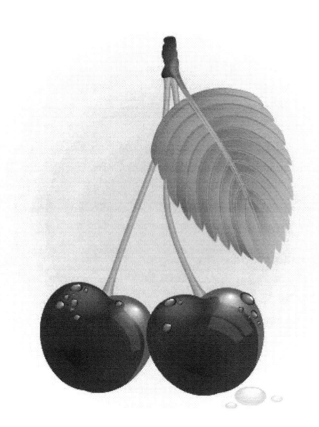

Blueberry Buckwheat Pancakes

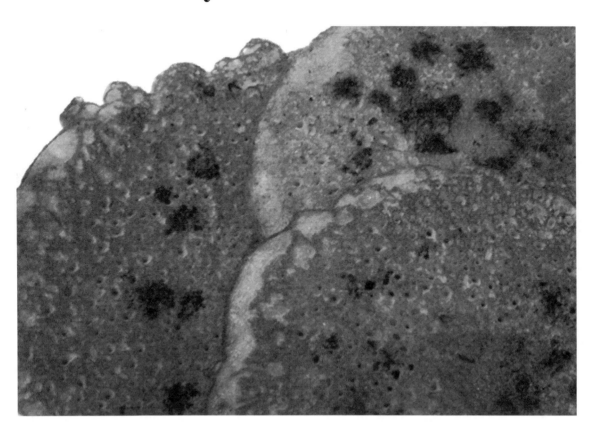

These pancakes are so good you won't be able to taste the difference between these and traditional ones (that is, if you ever ate ones made with regular buttermilk and eggs). This recipe lends itself to other types of fruit as well. Try small pieces of strawberries or mashing up some blackberries to give this delicacy a different taste. Have fun experimenting!

Ingredients

- ¼ cup rolled oats

- 1½ cups buckwheat flour

- 1 tablespoon baking powder

- 2 teaspoons sugar

- ½ teaspoon cinnamon

- ¼ teaspoon ground allspice

- ½ cup pecans or walnuts, chopped (optional. Toasted tastes great, too)

- 2¼ cups vegan buttermilk

- ½ cup blueberries

- 2 tablespoons coconut oil

- Your favorite topping for pancakes

Directions

1. In a large bowl, combine the oats, flour, baking powder, sugar, cinnamon, allspice, and nuts (if using) until thoroughly blended

2. Add the buttermilk and mix GENTLY just until dry ingredients are wet. Do not over mix!

3. Gently stir in the blueberries

4. Using a griddle or large frying pan on your stovetop, melt the coconut oil

5. When the pan is really hot, pour between 1/4 cup and 1/2 cup of batter on the griddle

6. Once the pancake batter begins to bubble and the sides dry out (about 4 minutes), flip the pancake and brown on the other side (about 3 minutes)

7. Continue in this manner, adding additional coconut oil to your pan if necessary, until the batter is used up

8. Enjoy with your favorite topping--like pure maple syrup or fruit preserves

Makes 2 to 3 servings

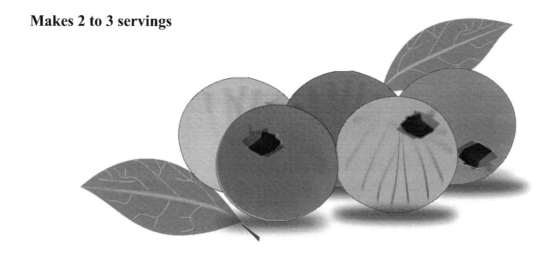

Lunch Recipes

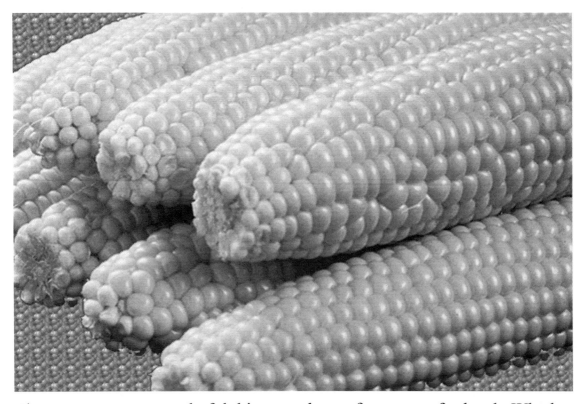

There are so many wonderful things to choose from to eat for lunch. Whether it is leftover dinner foods you heat up for lunch, savor a delicious salad, or enjoy a sandwich with veggies like tomatoes and cucumbers, you will find lunch ideas to please the masses.

While some of these recipes require some time, they are easy to make when you are not in a hurry. If you are, pick recipes that don't require much time. Otherwise, you can always use some of these delicious recipes as a great addition to your dinner meal menus.

Tasty Potato Salad

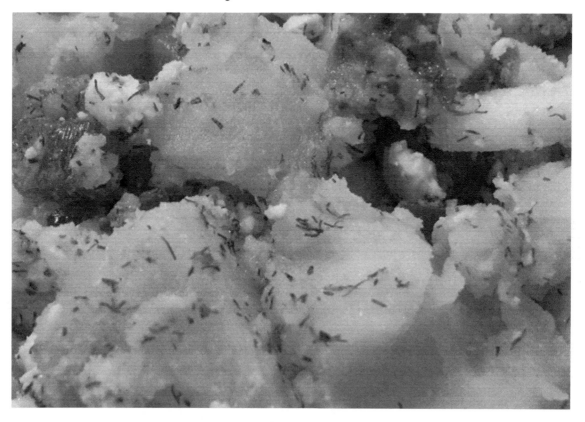

Traditional favorites like potato salad can still be enjoyed on a plant-based diet with just a few changes. Enjoy!

Ingredients:

- 3 pounds potatoes, peeled and cut into 1-inch chunks

- 1 tablespoon spicy mustard

- 2 tablespoons olive oil

- ¼ cup apple cider vinegar

- 1½ teaspoon salt

- ½ teaspoon pepper

- ½ cup milk alternative

- ¾ cup vegan mayonnaise

- 2 celery stalks, chopped

- 2 green onions, chopped

- ½ red onion, chopped

- 3 Roma tomatoes, chopped

- 2 tablespoons chives

Directions:

1. In a medium saucepan, place cut-up potatoes

2. Fill the saucepan with enough water to cover the potatoes

3. Bring to a boil over high heat

4. Once a boil is reached, turn the heat down to low and simmer for 10 minutes. The potatoes are done when a fork pokes easily into them

5. When the potatoes are done, remove them from the heat and drain the water from them

6. Allow the potatoes to cool

7. While the potatoes have cooled, combine the mustard, oil, vinegar, salt and pepper in a large bowl

8. Now place the potatoes into the large bowl containing the dressing and stir gently

9. In a separate bowl, thoroughly combine the milk and the mayonnaise together

10. Now add the celery, both kinds of onions, chopped tomatoes and chives to the milk mixture

11. Pour the milk mixture in with the potatoes and dressing and mix until thoroughly blended

12. Eat immediately or refrigerate if you like your potato salad chilled

Makes 6 to 8 servings

Veggie-Bobs on the Grill

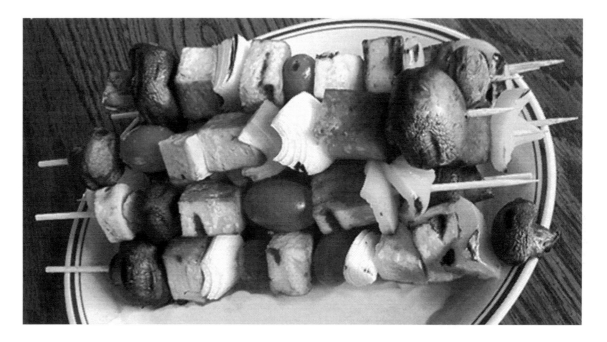

Vegetables take on a whole new flavor and sweetness when you grill them. Try these for your next gathering of family and friends.

Ingredients:

- 8 long wooden skewers

- 2 blocks extra-firm tofu

- 4 bell peppers

- 2 medium onions

- 1 package button mushrooms

- 2 tablespoons olive oil

- ½ teaspoon salt

- ¼ teaspoon pepper

Directions:

1. Before you begin, soak the wooden skewers in hot water for 45 minutes.

2. While they are soaking, heat up your grill to a medium heat setting.

3. Squeeze out as much liquid from the tofu as you can

4. Now pat them dry and cut into bite-sized cubes

5. Now, cut up the bell peppers into 1-inch pieces

6. Cut the onions into wedges—about 8 per onion

7. Wipe off the mushroom buttons of any visible dirt

8. Once the skewers have soaked, begin placing the vegetables on the skewers in an alternating pattern.

9. Lay the skewers onto a platter or foil.

10. Brush on the oil and then sprinkle salt, pepper, and any other favorite seasoning you like onto them.

11. Place the skewers on the hot grill.

12. Cover and grill the vegetables for 8 to 10 minutes or until they are cooked the way you like.

Makes 8 servings

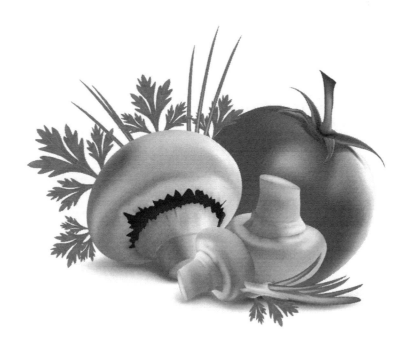

Broccoli Soup

Ingredients:

- 1 celery stalk, sliced

- 1 carrot, peeled and thinly sliced

- 1 clove garlic, minced

- 1 small onion, chopped

- ½ cup vegetable stock

- ½ teaspoon dried marjoram

- ¼ teaspoon dried basil

- 2 cups milk alternative

- 2 cups chopped broccoli

- ½ cup pasta (elbow or orzo)

- 1 cup Tofutti® sour cream

Directions:

1. In a soup pot or Dutch oven, combine the celery, carrot, garlic, onion, stock, marjoram, and basil

2. Bring this mixture to a boil

3. Reduce to a simmer and cover

4. Cook for approximately 10 minutes

5. Now add in the milk and broccoli and bring back to a boil again

6. Lower the heat and cook until the broccoli is tender

7. Remove the soup from the heat and carefully puree in a blender or food processor

8. Return the puree to the soup pot and add the pasta

9. Cook until the pasta is done and the soup is heated through

10. Add salt and pepper to your liking

11. Serve and use sour cream as a topping if desired

Makes 2 servings

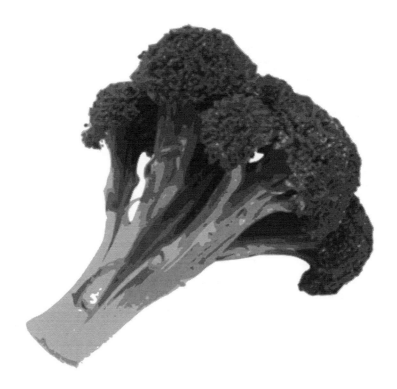

Summer Salad

Ingredients:

- ½ teaspoon spicy mustard

- 1 garlic clove, peeled and minced

- ⅓ cup balsamic vinegar

- ⅓ cup olive oil

- 4 large ripe tomatoes, diced

- 1 cucumber, peeled and diced

- 1 cup small pieces of broccoli florets

- 1 cup small pieces of cauliflower

- Salt and pepper to taste

- 1 red onion, peeled, halved, cut into slices, then separated into pieces

- 4 ounces vegan feta cheese, crumbled (page 81)

- 1 bunch fresh basil, chopped

Directions:

1. In a small bowl, combine the mustard, garlic, vinegar, and oil and mix thoroughly

2. In a medium-sized bowl combine the diced tomatoes, cucumber pieces, broccoli, cauliflower, and onion slices and mix gently

3. Pour the dressing over the vegetables

4. Sprinkle the vegan feta cheese crumbles over the vegetables

5. Top with the fresh basil

6. Chill if desired

You can also add some shredded lettuce with this salad if you want

Makes 2 to 3 servings

How to Make Vegan Feta Cheese

Here is a simple recipe for making your own feta cheese. It is good and doesn't take very long to make at all!

Ingredients

- 1 pound extra-firm tofu, drained and squeezed

- ¼ cup red wine vinegar

- 1/8 cup water

- 1 tablespoon lemon juice

- 4 teaspoons yellow miso paste

- 1 teaspoon salt

- 1 teaspoon dried oregano

- 2 teaspoons dried basil

- ¼ teaspoon dried rosemary

- 1 - 2 tablespoons nutritional yeast

Directions

1. In a medium bowl, break the drained tofu into small pieces

2. In a separate bowl, combine the vinegar, water, lemon juice, paste, salt, oregano, basil, and rosemary together using a hand whisk

3. Pour this mixture over the tofu and mix together using your hands. As you do, crumble up the tofu into small pieces

4. Allow the tofu to rest for 15 minutes

5. Now mix in 1 tablespoon of the nutritional yeast

6. Taste and decide if you want to add any more yeast

Black and Yellow Quesadillas

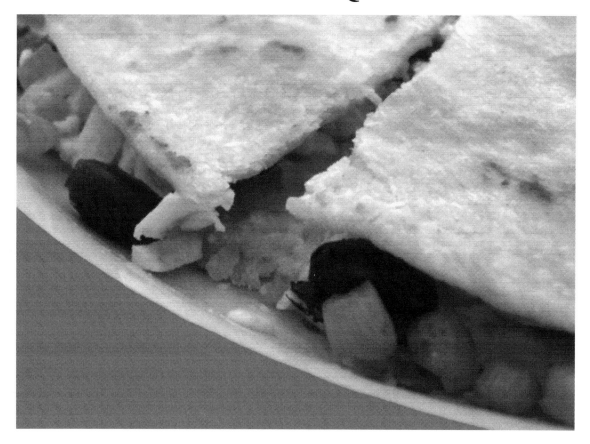

Quesadillas are so versatile! You can put so many wonderful foods and flavors between two tortilla shells to make meals special and delicious. Try this combination and see what you think.

Ingredients:

*   2 teaspoons coconut or olive oil

*   ½ small onion, chopped

*   1 (10 ounce) can whole kernel corn, drained

*   1 (15.5 ounce) can black beans, drained and rinsed

*   ¼ cup salsa

*   ¼ teaspoon red pepper flakes

- 2 tablespoons Earth Balance butter®

- 1 package of 8 inch flour tortillas

- 1½ cups vegan shredded cheese (your choice)

Directions:

1. Using a large frying pan, heat the oil over medium heat

2. Once heated, add the chopped onion and cook until tender

3. Add in the corn, black beans, salsa, and red pepper

4. Mix and heat the ingredients thoroughly

5. Place this mixture into a bowl and wipe out your pan so you can use it in the next step OR use another frying pan

6. Now, place 1 tablespoon of your butter into a large frying pan to melt it

7. Once the butter is hot, place a tortilla into the skillet

8. Sprinkle some of the cheese over the tortilla, followed by some of your bean mixture

9. Top all this with another tortilla

10. Cook until the bottom tortilla is golden brown

11. With two spatulas, flip the tortilla-sandwich as best you can

12. Cook the second tortilla until golden brown as well. This will allow the cheese inside to melt and will heat up the bean mixture, too

13. Continue this same process until you have used up your ingredients

Makes 5 quesadillas

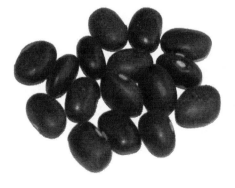

Greens, Tomatoes, and Pasta

Ingredients:

- 1 pound greens (mustard, collards, or turnip)—remove stems and chop
- 8 slices vegetarian bacon, diced
- 2 teaspoons coconut or olive oil
- ¼ teaspoon crushed red pepper
- 2 garlic cloves, minced
- 1 onion, chopped
- 1 (28-ounce) can diced tomatoes
- ¼ cup water
- 1 (8 ounce) box pasta shells
- Salt and pepper to taste
- ½ cup vegan Parmesan cheese (page 85)

Directions:

1. In a medium pot, fill about halfway with water and bring water to a boil
2. Add the greens to the boiling water and cook for approximately 10 minutes
3. Remove from your stovetop, pour into a strainer and rinse with cold water
4. Allow the greens to continue draining while you proceed with the next step
5. Rinse your pot you used for the greens OR use another pot filled halfway with water and bring it to a boil. This will be used for cooking the pasta
6. While the water is working its way to a boil, use a frying pan on your stovetop to cook the bacon pieces
7. Once they are finished cooking, remove the bacon pieces from the pan and set aside
8. Add the oil to your frying pan
9. Once the oil is heated, add the red pepper, garlic and onion
10. Cook until the onions are soft

11. Add the bacon pieces back into the pan, along with the tomatoes and water

12. Bring to a low boil and cook for approximately 20 minutes

13. After a few minutes, carefully use a potato masher or the edge of a large spoon to mash the tomatoes

14. By now, your water should be boiling, so add your pasta to the pot

15. Cook for approximately 10 minutes, stirring occasionally

16. Using a measuring cup, remove ¼ cup of the pasta water and set aside

17. When the pasta is finished cooking, drain it

18. Now add the pasta, collard greens, and pasta water to the tomato mixture

19. Heat ingredients thoroughly

20. Season with salt and pepper to your liking

21. When ready to serve, sprinkle the vegan Parmesan cheese on top

Makes 4 to 6 servings

How to Make Vegan Parmesan Cheese

As of this writing, there aren't a great deal of vegan Parmesan cheeses to choose from which is okay because here is a great recipe you can make quickly and enjoy anytime!

Ingredients
- 2 cups cashews, raw and unsalted
- 2 teaspoons salt
- ½ cup nutritional yeast

Directions
1. Using a food processor, place the cashews, salt, and yeast into the bowl and process until you have a smooth powder

2. That's it!

3. Store this in an airtight container in your refrigerator and enjoy it anytime you want some cheese on your pasta, pizza, or lasagna

Colorful Paninis

Paninis can make an ordinary sandwich, extraordinary just by heating up the sandwich with a Panini maker or using a griddle on your stovetop. We love making these at our house.

Ingredients:

- 2 red bell peppers (for color), cut in half and seeds removed

- 4 Portobello mushroom caps

- 1 cup balsamic vinaigrette

- 1 eggplant, peeled and sliced into ½ inch pieces

- 1 teaspoon onion powder

- 1 teaspoon garlic powder

- 2 teaspoons vegan Parmesan cheese (page 85)

- 8 slices focaccia bread

- ¼ cup vegan ranch dressing (page 87)

- 4 slices Tofutti® mozzarella cheese slices

- 4 slices vegan cheddar cheese slices (Vegan Gourmet® works well)

Directions:

1. Preheat your oven's broiler and place a rack about 6 inches from the heating element

2. Prepare a baking sheet covered in aluminum foil

3. Place the pepper halves down onto the foil with the cut sides down

4. Cook under the broiler until the skins have blistered—about 5 minutes

5. Remove the peppers and place in a bowl

6. Tightly cover the bowl with plastic wrap and allow to cool. This will make removing the skins easy

7. After the skins are removed, place in a sealed container and refrigerate for several hours or overnight

8. Once the peppers are in the refrigerator, place the mushroom caps into a Ziploc bag

9. Pour the vinaigrette over the caps and seal

10. Place mushrooms into the refrigerator along with the peppers and refrigerate several hours or overnight

11. When you are ready to make your paninis, preheat a double-sided indoor grill or Panini maker. (A griddle could be used if you don't have one of these)

12. Peel and slice your eggplant and sprinkle with onion powder and garlic powder

13. Remove the mushrooms from the marinade

14. Place the mushrooms on the preheated grill and cook for 5 minutes

15. Now cook the eggplant slices on the grill for approximately 5 minutes

16. Remove when cooked and sprinkle with Parmesan cheese

17. To assemble your Panini, spread each slice of focaccia with some ranch dressing

18. Place a slice of cheese on each piece of bread

19. Now place an eggplant slice, a roasted pepper, and a mushroom cap on each of 4 slices

20. Top with the remaining 4 slices of bread

21. Now place each sandwich on your grill or Panini maker

22. Cook until the cheeses are melted and the bread is toasted to a beautiful golden brown on each side

Makes 4 paninis

How to Make Vegan Ranch Dressing

Here is a great tasting recipe for ranch dressing you can make at home using easy-to-find ingredients. If you want to use it as a dip, just add a little bit of extra mayonnaise and a little less milk so its consistency is thicker.

Ingredients

- ½ cup milk alternative (nut, rice, or soy)

- 2 cups vegan mayonnaise

- 2 teaspoons garlic powder

- ½ teaspoon salt

- ½ teaspoon black pepper

- 2 teaspoons onion powder

- 4 teaspoons fresh chopped parsley

- ½ teaspoon dried dill

- 2 tablespoons apple cider vinegar

Directions

1. Place all your ingredients into a food processor or a blender and process until you have a creamy and smooth consistency

2. Keep refrigerated

Another way to make your own ranch dressing is to reconstitute the dry mix with the following:

Ingredients

- 1½ cup vegan mayonnaise

- 1 cup unsweetened nondairy milk

- 2 tablespoons dry ranch dressing mix

- 1 tablespoon vinegar

Directions

1. Combine all the ingredients together until it is a smooth consistency

2. Refrigerate

Makes about 2 cups of dressing

Pasta Salad with Veggies

Ingredients:

- 2 tablespoons red wine vinegar

- 3 tablespoons olive oil

- 1 teaspoon garlic powder

- 1 teaspoon spicy mustard

- Salt and pepper to taste

- ½ cup fresh mushrooms, chopped

- ½ cup onion, chopped

- ½ cup green bell pepper, chopped

- ½ cup yellow bell pepper, chopped

- 1 (8 ounce) package penne pasta

- 2 tablespoons vegan mayonnaise

- 2 tablespoons vegan Parmesan cheese (page 85)

Directions:

1. Preheat your oven broiler

2. Place a saucepan full of lightly salted water on the stovetop to bring it to a boil for the pasta

3. In a bowl, mix the vinegar, oil, garlic powder, mustard, salt, and pepper

4. Place the mushrooms, onion, and bell peppers on a baking sheet

5. Pour the oil and vinegar mixture over the vegetables

6. Broil the vegetables for 5 minutes, stirring occasionally, until they are lightly scorched

7. Remove from under the heat and allow them to cool

8. Add the pasta to boiling water and cook for 8 to 10 minutes

9. Drain and rinse with cold water to cool

10. Place the vegetables, pasta, and mayonnaise in a large bowl

11. Toss gently

12. Top with the Parmesan cheese when serving

Makes 4 servings

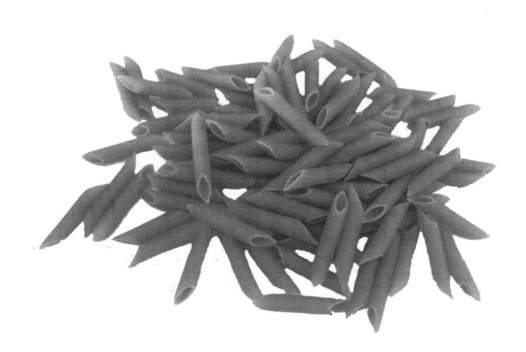

Grilled Cheese with Apple

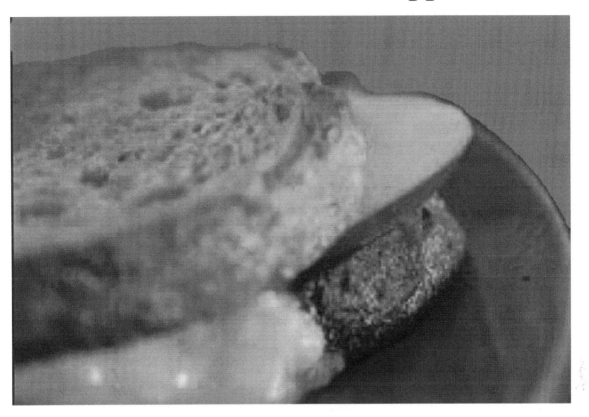

Grilled cheese is a standard lunch in many households, so why not take a favorite and add a little something special to it. By using some nut butter and thin slices of apples, you are bound to create a new favorite at your house!

Ingredients:

- Earth Balance Butter® for frying

- 2 slices whole wheat bread

- 2 tablespoons of your favorite nut butter

- 2 slices vegan cheddar cheese (try Vegan Gourmet®)

- ½ apple thinly sliced

Directions:

1. Place a frying pan or skillet over medium heat

2. Melt a small amount of butter in the skillet

3. Now spread some nut butter on one side of your bread

4. Place the bread, nut butter side UP on the skillet

5. Put one slice of cheese on the bread

6. Now sprinkle apple pieces on top of the cheese

7. Place the second piece of cheese on top of the apples

8. Put the second piece of bread on top of the cheese—nut buttered side DOWN

9. Once the bottom piece of bread has browned, flip the sandwich over to brown the second side

10. Once your cheese has melted, your sandwich is ready to be enjoyed

Makes 1 sandwich

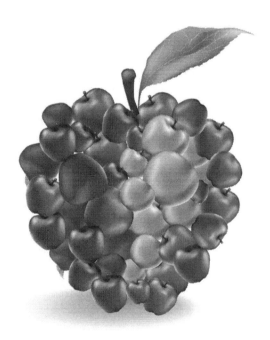

Vegetarian Chili

Ingredients:

- 1 (28 ounce) can diced tomatoes with juice

- 1 (15 ounce) can white beans, drained

- 1 (15 ounce) can kidney beans, with liquid

- 1 small onion, diced

- 2 tablespoons ranch dressing mix

- 2 tablespoons taco seasoning mix (page 94)

- 1 (12 ounce) package vegetarian burger crumbles

- 1 (8 ounce) package vegan shredded cheese

Directions:

1. In a large saucepan, pour the tomatoes, white beans, kidney beans, onion, ranch mix, and taco mix and cook over medium heat

2. Bring mixture to a boil

3. Once a boil is reached, reduce the heat to low and add the veggie crumbles

4. Continue cooking until heated through

5. Top with the shredded cheese and serve

Makes 4 to 6 servings

How to Make Ranch Dressing (dry mix)

Ingredients

- 1 tablespoon dried parsley

- 1 teaspoon onion powder

- 1 teaspoon minced onion

- 1 teaspoon dried dill weed

- ½ teaspoon garlic powder

- 1 teaspoon dried chives

- 1 teaspoon salt

- ¼ teaspoon black pepper

Directions

1. In a small bowl, combine all the ingredients together

2. Store in an airtight container until you are ready to use it

How to Make Taco Seasoning Mix (dry)

Ingredients

- 2 tablespoons chili powder

- 1 tablespoon ground cumin

- 1 tablespoon garlic powder

- 2 teaspoons dried oregano

- 1 tablespoons onion powder

- 1½ teaspoons arrowroot powder

- 2 teaspoons paprika

- ½ teaspoon crushed red pepper flakes, to taste

- 1½ teaspoons brown sugar

- 2 teaspoons salt

Directions

1. Combine all the ingredients together and mix

2. Store in an airtight container until ready to use

Fruity Yogurt Salad

Ingredients:

- ¼ cup honey

- 1 cup soy yogurt

- ¼ teaspoon celery seed

- 2 tablespoons spicy mustard

- Handful of romaine lettuce pieces

- Handful of baby spinach leaves

- ½ fresh pineapple cubes

- ½ cup raspberries

- ¼ cup sliced almonds

Directions:

1. In a small bowl, combine the honey, yogurt, celery seed, and mustard and mix thoroughly

2. In a medium-sized bowl, place the romaine pieces, baby spinach, pineapple, and raspberries and mix gently

3. Now pour the dressing over the lettuce and fruit and stir to distribute the dressing throughout your salad

4. Top with the almonds when ready to serve

Makes 1 serving

Stuffed Peppers

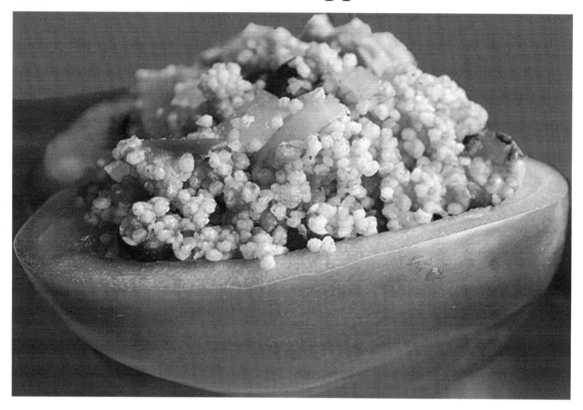

Try this delicious lunch or dinner menu item using couscous instead of the traditional rice option. So good and healthy!

Ingredients:

- 1 tablespoon coconut oil

- 1 small onion, peeled and chopped

- 2 large bell peppers (any color), seeded and halved

- 3 ounces couscous

- 2/3 cup boiling water

- 2 ounces dried tomatoes, snipped into small pieces

- 8 black olives, roughly chopped

- 1 ounce pine nuts, toast if desired

- 2 ounces vegan feta cheese (page 81)

- 2 tablespoons fresh basil, chopped

Directions:

1. Preheat your oven to 400 degrees F

2. In a small frying pan on your stovetop, heat up the coconut oil

3. Now place the onion pieces into the frying pan and sauté until tender—about 5 to 6 minutes

4. Remove from the stovetop and set aside

5. As the onions are cooking, place the bell peppers on a microwave-safe plate and cook on medium for 5 minutes. This will soften the peppers

6. Now place the peppers on a cookie sheet, cut side up

7. Pour the couscous into a bowl and cover with ⅔ cup boiling water

8. Stir, then cover the bowl and let it stand for 10 minutes

9. Stir the couscous with a fork to break it up

10. Now add the onions, tomatoes, olives, pine nuts, cheese, and basil and mix thoroughly

11. Place equal amounts of the couscous mixture into the bell pepper halves

12. Put the stuffed peppers into the oven for 10 to 15 minutes

13. Serve hot

Makes 4 servings

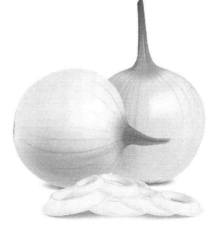

Pasta Primavera

Ingredients:

- 1 bunch fresh basil

- ½ cup olive oil plus 2 tablespoons

- 3 cups vegetable broth

- 2 garlic cloves

- 1 bunch green onions, chopped

- 1 large leek, chopped, washed, dark parts removed

- 1 bunch asparagus, leave tips whole, dice the stalks

- 1 cup green peas

- Salt and pepper to taste

- 2 green zucchini, diced

- ½ cup vegan Parmesan cheese (page 85)

- 1 pound thin spaghetti

Directions:

1. Fill a large saucepan with water and bring it to a boil

2. Dip the basil leaves into the boiling water for 5 seconds, then place in a bowl with ice water to stop the leaves from cooking any further. Keep the water boiling for cooking the pasta in a few minutes

3. Remove the basil leaves from the stems and place them into a blender with ½ cup oil, 1 cup of vegetable broth, and the garlic

4. Blend until smooth

5. In another large saucepan, place the remaining 2 tablespoons of oil and heat

6. Place the green onions and leeks into the pan and cook for approximately 10 minutes

7. Add the asparagus, peas, salt, pepper, zucchini, and the remaining 2 cups of broth

8. Increase the heat to high and cook vegetables for 7 to 8 minutes

9. Remove from the heat

10. Now add the pasta to the boiling water and cook according to package directions

11. When tender, pour into a colander to drain

12. Transfer the pasta to a large serving bowl

13. Now pour the vegetables and basil mixture over the pasta

14. Toss to mix well

15. Sprinkle on the cheese and mix gently

16. Cover briefly to allow the pasta to absorb some of the juices, then serve

17. Garnish with more cheese, salt and pepper if desired

Makes 4 to 6 servings

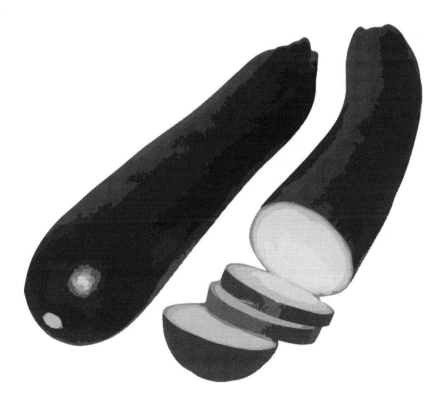

Beans and Rice Enchiladas with a Kick

This recipe is a great crowd pleaser—even for people who are not plant-based eaters! These are not only good for lunch, but will work great for a gathering of friends and family.

Ingredients:

- 2 tablespoons coconut oil

- 1 (4 ounce) can green chilies

- 1 yellow bell pepper, chopped

- 1 red bell pepper, chopped

- 1 onion, chopped

- 2 garlic cloves, minced

- 10 (8 inch) flour tortillas

- 1 cup brown rice, cooked (leftover from a previous meal)

- 1 (15 ounce) can black beans, drained

- 1 (15 ounce) can pinto beans, drained

- ¼ teaspoon hot pepper sauce

- 1 teaspoon ground cumin

- ½ teaspoon chili powder

- 1 cup vegan shredded cheese (your choice)

- 1 cup of your favorite salsa

Directions:

1. Preheat your oven to 350 degrees F

2. Lightly grease a 9 x 13 inch baking pan and set aside

3. On your stovetop, take a large frying pan and add the coconut oil

4. Add the chilies, bell peppers, onion, and garlic and sauté until vegetables are tender--approximately 10 minutes

5. While the vegetables are cooking, wrap the tortillas in foil and place them into your preheated oven for about 10 minutes. This will make them warm and pliable

6. Once the vegetables are tender, add the rice, black beans and pinto beans into the frying pan

7. Now add the hot pepper sauce, cumin, and chili powder and mix well

8. Heat for about 8 to 10 minutes, until any excess liquids have been absorbed into the rice

9. Unwrap the tortilla and spoon about ½ cup of the mixture into the center of each tortilla and roll up the tortilla

10. Taking your baking pan and place each tortilla seam side DOWN into the dish

11. Sprinkle the tortillas with the shredded cheese

12. Place the baking dish into your preheated oven and bake until the cheese melts—about 10 minutes

13. Once the tortillas are done, serve with a topping of your favorite salsa

Makes 10 enchiladas

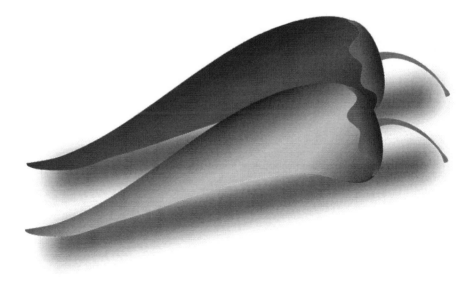

Toasted Corn Salad with Beans and Peppers

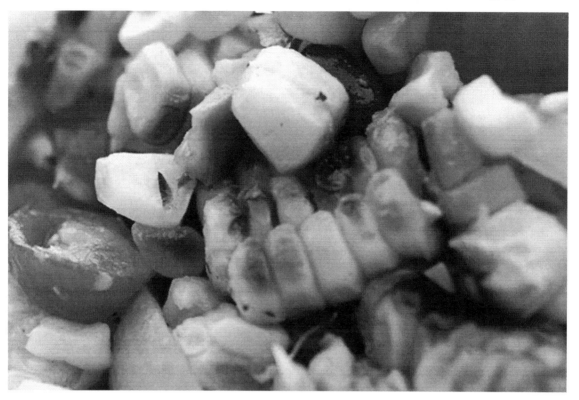

Ingredients:

Dressing

- ¼ cup olive oil

- ¼ cup vegan mayonnaise

- ½ teaspoon sugar

- ¼ cup red wine vinegar

- 1 garlic clove, minced

- ½ teaspoon pepper

- ½ teaspoon salt

Salad

- 2 tablespoons olive oil

- 4 cups fresh corn (or frozen that has been thawed)

- 1 (15 ounce) can black beans, drained

- 1 cup cherry tomatoes, diced

- ½ green bell pepper, diced

- 1 small onion

- Cayenne to taste

- Salt and pepper to taste

Directions:

1. In a small bowl, add the oil, mayonnaise, sugar, vinegar, garlic, pepper, and salt and blend thoroughly

2. Set aside

3. In a large skillet over medium heat, add the oil and heat.

4. When the oil is hot, add the corn and cook for 8 minutes. You want the kernels to be lightly toasted

5. Remove from the heat and add to a medium-sized mixing bowl

6. Add the black beans to the corn

7. Now add in the tomatoes, green pepper, onion, cayenne, salt, pepper and dressing you made earlier to the corn and beans and combine thoroughly

8. Cover the bowl and refrigerate for at least an hour

9. Once it reaches your desired temperature, serve and enjoy

Makes 4 to 6 servings

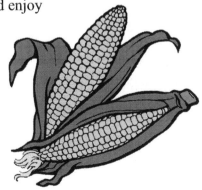

Red and Green Salad

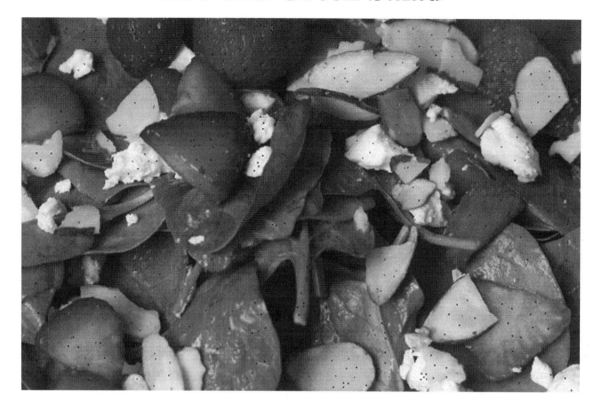

Not only is this salad declicious and easy to make, but it is really pretty, too!

Ingredients:

- 3 tablespoons sugar

- ½ cup sliced almonds

- ¾ tablespoon poppy seeds

- ¼ cup sugar

- ¾ cup red wine vinegar

- ⅓ cup olive oil

- 2 tablespoons mustard

- ¾ teaspoon salt

- 2 (6 ounce) bags baby spinach leaves

- 1 (12 ounce) bag vegan shredded cheese

- 2 cups fresh strawberries OR dried cranberries

Directions:

1. In a small skillet over medium heat, cook the sugar and almonds until the sugar is melted all over the almonds. This should take about 3 to 4 minutes

2. Remove the almonds from the pan and spread out onto waxed paper or parchment paper to cool

3. In a small bowl, whisk together the poppy seeds, sugar, vinegar, oil, mustard, and salt

4. Now, in a large bowl, place the spinach, cheese, strawberries or dried cranberries

5. Toss gently to mix

6. Sprinkle the almonds over the lettuce mix

7. Now drizzle the dressing over the top of the salad and toss

8. Serve immediately

Makes 4 to 6 servings

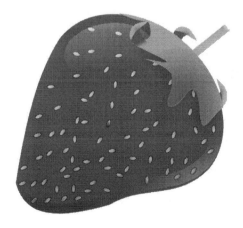

Curried Brown Rice with Lentils

This makes a very filling lunch or main dinner dish when served over wilted spinach

Ingredients:

- 1 tablespoon Earth Balance Butter®
- 1 cup brown rice
- 1 tablespoon curry powder
- 4¼ cups water
- 4 garlic cloves, peeled
- 1 cinnamon stick
- 1 cup brown lentils
- ½ teaspoon salt
- 4 slices fresh ginger, each slice about ⅛ inch thick
- 4 scallions, sliced

Directions:

1. Preheat your oven to 350 degrees F
2. On your stovetop, melt the butter in a large oven-proof Dutch oven
3. Add the rice and cook until lightly toasted. This should take about 2 minutes
4. Now add the curry powder and cook for an additional 20 to 30 seconds—until the mixture becomes fragrant
5. Now add the water
6. Stir in the garlic, cinnamon, lentils, salt, and ginger slices
7. Cover the pot and transfer it to your preheated oven
8. Bake for 1 hour until the rice and lentils are tender and the water is absorbed
9. Fluff with a fork while removing the cinnamon stick and ginger slices
10. Serve with a garnish of the scallions

Makes 4 (1/2 cup) servings

Light Eggplant Parmesan

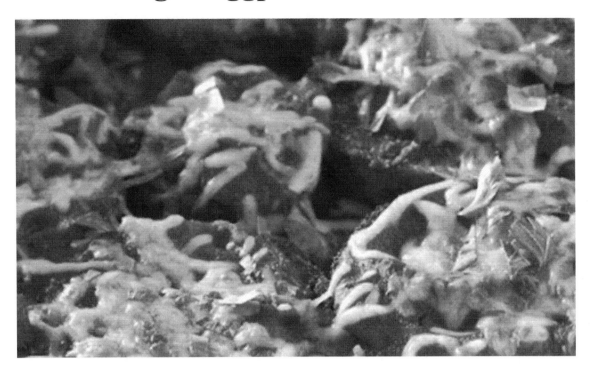

This dish is more involved than many of the other lunch dishes so you will probably want to make it for lunch or dinner on the weekends. Whenever you decide to make it, be assured that it is definitely worth your time and effort. It is scrumptious!

Ingredients:

- 2 large eggplants, peeled and cut into ½ inch thick slices

- 4 tablespoons olive or coconut oil

- ¼ cup non-dairy shredded cheese (your choice)

- ½ cup vegan Parmesan cheese (page 85)

- ¾ cup vegan ricotta cheese (page 109)

- 2 garlic cloves, sliced

- 3 cups tomato sauce

- ½ cup water

- Additional ½ cup vegan Parmesan cheese (page 85)

- ¾ cup breadcrumbs

- Salt and pepper to taste

- 1 bunch fresh basil, chopped (optional)

Directions:

1. Take the 12 widest eggplant slices and set them aside

2. Now dice the remaining eggplant slices and reserve for later

3. Add 1 tablespoon of oil into your frying pan and heat

4. Add the garlic and cook until it begins to sizzle

5. Add the diced eggplant you reserved earlier and cook for 5 minutes

6. Add in the tomato sauce, water, salt, and pepper

7. Turn heat to low and cook for 15 to 20 minutes

8. Preheat your oven to 375 degrees F

9. In another frying pan, add 1 tablespoon of oil and heat

10. Once heated, place the eggplant slices into the oil and cook 3 minutes on each side

11. After the slices are cooked, place them on paper towels to drain

12. As the slices are cooling, take a small bowl and mix the 3 cheeses

13. Once the sauce is finished cooking, pour half of the sauce into the bottom of the dish

14. Place 6 of the eggplant slices on top of the sauce

15. Spoon the cheese mixture on to these eggplant slices

16. Now place the other 6 slices on top of the cheese mixture

17. Now pour the remaining sauce over the eggplant

18. In a small bowl, combine the remaining 2 tablespoons of oil, Parmesan cheese, and breadcrumbs and mix

19. Spread over the eggplant

20. Place the baking dish in your preheated oven and cook for 45 minutes

21. Once the eggplant is bubbling and crisp looking on the top, remove from the oven

22. Allow the dish to sit for 15 minutes before serving

How to Make Vegan Ricotta Cheese

If you have trouble finding non-dairy ricotta cheese or just want to make your own so you know what is in it, here is a recipe I think you will enjoy making.

Ingredients
- 1 (12.3 ounce) package extra-firm tofu
- ¾ teaspoon red wine vinegar
- 1½ teaspoons extra-virgin olive oil
- 4½ teaspoons fresh lemon juice
- ¾ teaspoon shallot, finely chopped
- ¾ teaspoon garlic, minced
- ¾ teaspoon fresh parsley, chopped
- ¾ teaspoon fresh basil, chopped
- 1½ teaspoons nutritional yeast flakes

Directions
1. Squeeze out any water from the tofu then either crumble it up with your hands or run it through a potato ricer and place in a large bowl

2. Add each of the other ingredients and mix thoroughly. This should result in a ricotta cheese consistency

Makes 2 cups

Nutty Pesto Sandwiches

Ingredients:

- ¼ cup cashew pieces

- ½ cup fresh basil

- ¼ cup olive oil

- ½ teaspoon black pepper

- Salt to taste

- 12 black olives, chopped

- 8 whole wheat bread slices, lightly buttered

- 8 vegan cheese slices (your choice)

- 1 - 2 tomatoes, sliced

Directions:

1. Begin by placing the cashews, basil, oil, pepper and salt into a blender

2. Blend until smooth

3. Empty the mixture into a bowl

4. Now add the chopped olives

5. Take the bread slices and remove the crusts, if desired

6. Take the olive mixture and spread it equally onto 4 of the slices of bread

7. Place two cheese slices and a tomato slice on top of the olive mixture

8. Put a second piece of bread on top

9. Serve immediately

Makes 4 sandwiches

Veggies in the Rye

Ingredients

- 4 pieces dark rye bread

- 4 tablespoons non-dairy cream cheese

- 1 tomato, sliced

- 1 avocado, sliced

- 1 cucumber, peeled and sliced

- 2 small kale leaves, stem removed

- 2 small handfuls of sprouts (alfalfa, broccoli, etc.)

- 2 teaspoons balsamic vinegar

- 2 teaspoons olive oil

- 1 teaspoon garlic, minced

Directions

1. Begin by spreading the 4 slices of bread with the cream cheese

2. Now add a couple of slices of tomato and several slices of avocado to two of the slices

3. Place cucumber slices on top of the tomato and avocado

4. Put one kale leaf over the cucumber slices

5. Add some sprouts to cover the veggies

6. In a small bowl, combine the vinegar, oil, and garlic and mix

7. Gently pour some of the dressing over the top of the veggies

8. Place the remaining two slices of bread on top of each sandwich

Yummy!

Makes 2 sandwiches

Bagels on the Go

Here is a sandwich that is easy to make and goes where you go--a perfect sandwich to take to work or school, it will definitely get you revved up for the remaining part of your day

Ingredients

- 1 bagel (multigrain will give you a nutty taste)
- 2 tablespoons non-dairy cream cheese
- 2 slices of vegan cheddar cheese
- ¼ cup shredded carrot pieces
- 2 dill pickle slices
- 1 lettuce leaf

Directions

1. Slice the bagel in half carefully
2. Spread the cream cheese on each half of your bagel
3. Assemble the rest of your bagel to your liking, then place the top on your bagel

Makes 1 sandwich

How to Make Vegan Cheddar Cheese

Here is an easy way to make your own cheddar cheese. It is incredibly versatile and you can add ingredients to your liking after you make it a time or two.

Ingredients

- 4 tablespoons fresh lemon juice
- ¼ teaspoon dry mustard
- ½ teaspoon spicy mustard
- ½ teaspoon salt

- ½ cup cashew pieces

- 2 teaspoons onion powder

- 1/8 teaspoon cayenne pepper

- 1/3 cup nutritional yeast powder

- ¼ teaspoon garlic powder

- 5 tablespoons agar-agar flakes OR 5 teaspoons of powdered agar-agar

- 1½ cups water

Directions

1. Using a non-stick cooking spray, lightly grease a small 3" x 7" loaf pan. This will be the shape of your cheese when you are done

2. Into a blender, combine the lemon juice, dry mustard, spicy mustard, salt, cashews, onion powder, cayenne pepper, yeast, and garlic powder. Do NOT process yet

3. Using a small saucepan on your stovetop, combine the agar-agar with the water and process over medium heat

4. While stirring frequently, bring the mixture to a boil

5. Now reduce the heat, but keep a gentle boil going for approximately 5 minutes, making sure all the agar gets dissolved

6. Now pour the agar water carefully into the blender with the other ingredients and place the lid on top

7. Blend on the highest speed for approximately 1 minute

8. Turn off the blender, scrape down the sides with a rubber spatula, then replace the top and blend on high again for another minute

9. Using your prepared loaf pan, carefully pour the mixture in

10. Put your loaf pan into your refrigerator and allow the cheese to chill until it is a firm consistency

11. Once it is firm, you are ready to slice your cheese and enjoy

Makes one 7-inch cheese log

AAA Salad

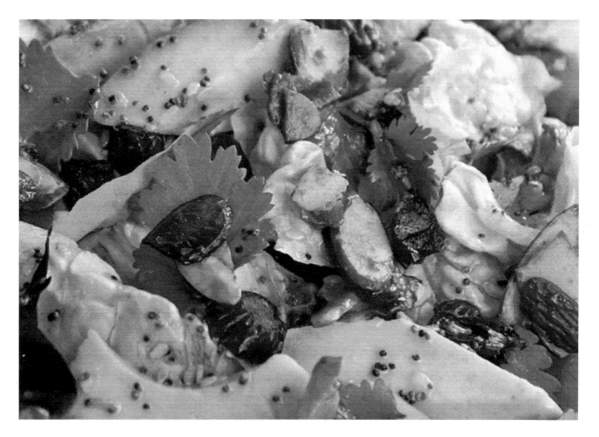

This is a delicious salad to enjoy at home or to take along with you wherever you go.

Ingredients

- 1 tablespoon olive oil

- 1 garlic clove, peeled and minced

- ¼ teaspoon salt

- 1/8 teaspoon ground pepper

- 1 tablespoon dried dill

- 1 tablespoon lemon juice

- 2 tablespoons poppy seeds

- 2 cups lettuce (your choice)

- ¼ onion, chopped

- 1 avocado, peeled, seed removed, sliced or cut into small chunks

- 1 Granny Smith apple, cored and cut into small chunks (peel if desired)

- ¼ cup sliced almonds

- ¼ dried cranberries

Directions

1. Using a small bowl, mix together the oil, garlic, salt, pepper, dill, lemon juice, and poppy seeds thoroughly

2. In another bowl, add the lettuce, onion, avocado, apple chunks, nuts and cranberries and toss gently

3. Pour the dressing over the top of the greens, toss, and eat

Makes 1 to 2 servings

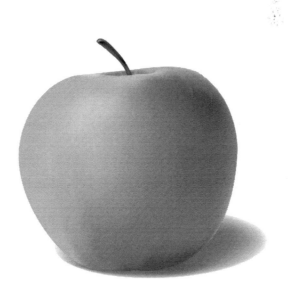

Pizza for One

Whether you enjoy this pizza at home or decide to take it to work, it is delicious anytime, anywhere

Ingredients

- 1 tablespoon coconut oil for frying

- 1 small flour or corn tortilla

- ¼ sweet bell pepper, chopped

- ¼ small red onion, chopped

- 1 garlic clove, peeled and minced

- 3 to 4 mushroom buttons, sliced or chopped

- ½ tomato, thinly sliced

- ¼ teaspoon dried oregano

- ¼ teaspoon dried basil

- 1/3 to ½ cup non-dairy shredded Mozzarella cheese

Directions

1. Preheat your oven to 400 degrees F

2. Placing a small frying pan on your stovetop, heat up the oil

3. Place your tortilla into the hot oil and fry on both sides so that both sides have a nice brown color

4. Remove from heat

5. Drain on paper towels if necessary

6. Take a small baking sheet and line with foil

7. Place the cooked tortilla on the foil

8. Returning to your stovetop and place a little more coconut oil in your pan if necessary for additional frying and heat

9. Place the bell pepper, onion, garlic, and mushroom into the frying pan and sauté until tender--about 6 to 7 minutes

10. Place the cooked vegetables on top of your tortilla

11. Put the tomato slices on next

12. Now sprinkle on the oregano and basil

13. Top with the shredded cheese

14. Place your pizza into your preheated oven and bake for 8 to 10 minutes--until the cheese has melted

15. Remove from the oven and cut into serving slices

Makes 1 pizza

Note: If you will be eating your pizza at work, you can assemble the pizza at home and cook it in a toaster oven when lunchtime arrives

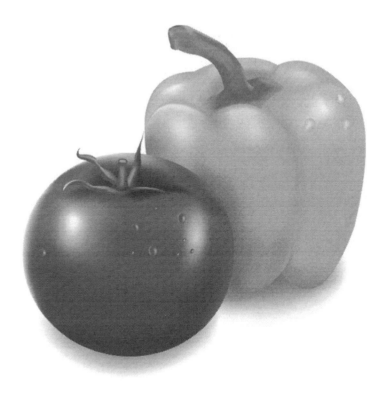

Delicious Homemade Soup

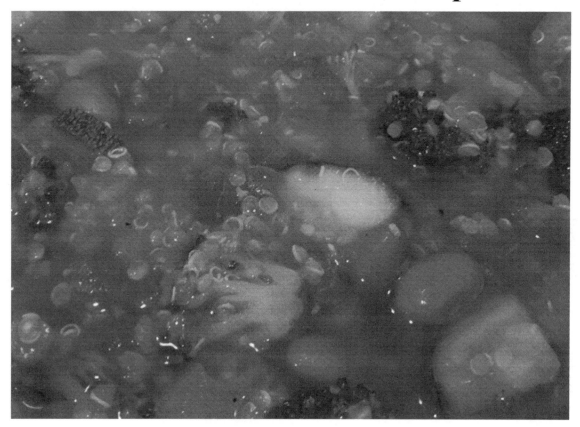

Here is a delicious soup that will warm you down to your toenails. It takes a little while to cook on your stovetop or in your crockpot, but once you do, it is very easy to reheat, too. While this recipe makes 2 servings, feel free to double and triple it to feed your whole crew or to enjoy when friends come over.

Ingredients

- 2 cups vegetable broth

- ¾ cup quinoa, uncooked

- 2 cups small broccoli florets

- 1 cup baby carrots OR 1 carrot, peeled and sliced

- 1 celery stalk, sliced

- ½ zucchini, cubed

- ½ small onion, chopped

- 1 (15 ounce) can diced tomato

- ½ teaspoon salt

- ¼ teaspoon black pepper

- ½ teaspoon garlic powder

- ½ teaspoon marjoram

- ¼ teaspoon paprika

- ¼ teaspoon thyme

- ¼ teaspoon dried parsley

Directions

1. On your stovetop in a medium-sized saucepan, place all the ingredients.

2. Bring to a boil

3. Now cover and lower the temperature so it can slowly simmer for about one hour

4. Your soup is done when the quinoa is cooked through and the vegetables are tender.

Makes 2 servings

Note: You could also make this dish with brown or wild rice instead of quinoa.

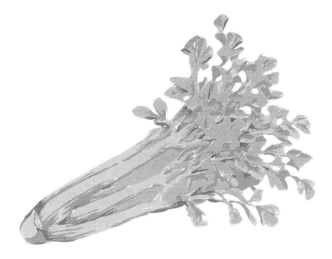

Mighty Good Quesadillas

Ingredients

- 1 tablespoon coconut or olive oil

- ¼ onion, finely chopped

- 1 garlic clove, peeled and minced

- 1 cup corn, canned or frozen (drain if using canned)

- 2 (8 ounce) cans vegetarian refried beans

- ¼ cup favorite salsa

- 1 tablespoon honey

- ½ teaspoon crushed red pepper

- 8 (8 inch) flour tortillas

- 1 cup vegan Monterey Jack cheese, shredded

- ½ cup vegan extra sharp cheddar cheese, shredded

- ¼ cup non-dairy sour cream

Directions

1. Preheat your oven to 350 degrees F

2. In a large saucepan, heat the oil over medium heat

3. Add the onion and garlic to the pan and sauté about 2 minutes until tender

4. Now stir in the corn and beans

5. Add in 2 tablespoons of salsa, the honey, and pepper flakes

6. Cook until heated through--about 3 minutes

7. On a baking sheet, place 4 of your tortillas

8. Cover each one evenly with the cheeses

9. Now evenly divide the warm bean mixture among the 4 tortillas

10. Cover these with the other 4 tortillas

11. Place the baking sheet into your preheated oven and bake until golden brown and when the cheeses have melted--about 15 minutes

12. Cut in quesadillas into wedges and serve with remaining salsa, the guacamole, and sour cream

Makes 4 quesadillas

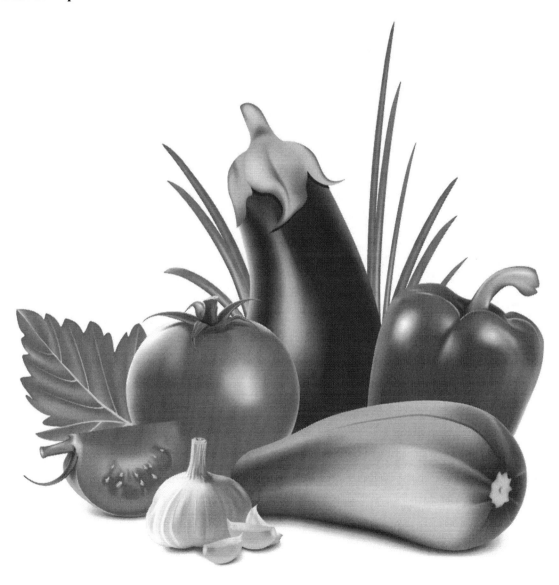

Macaroni Salad

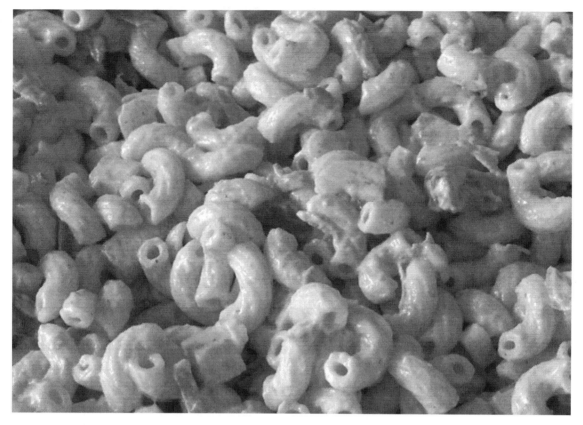

After you make this salad a time or two, consider adding some vegetarian ham to it, or serve it up with some crackers. You can do many things with this classic.

Ingredients

- 1 tablespoon yellow mustard

- 1 tablespoon fresh lemon juice

- 1 tablespoon vinegar

- 1 cup vegan mayonnaise

- ½ teaspoon salt

- ¼ teaspoon black pepper

- 1 teaspoon sugar

- 1 (8 ounce) bag macaroni (your choice of shape)

- ½ small onion, peeled and chopped

- 1 sweet bell pepper, chopped

- 2 Roma tomatoes, chopped

Directions

1. Place a pot of water on your stovetop to boil

2. While you are waiting for the water to boil, begin the rest of your salad

3. In a separate bowl, combine the mustard, lemon juice, vinegar, vegan mayonnaise, salt, pepper, and sugar thoroughly

4. Once the water is boiling, add the macaroni and cook according to package directions

5. Now add the onion, pepper, and tomato to the bowl and mix in with the other ingredients

6. Using a strainer, drain off the water from the macaroni once it is finished cooking

7. Add the macaroni to your other ingredients

8. Mix thoroughly, cover, and place in your refrigerator

9. Once it is chilled, you are ready to enjoy eating it

Makes 4 servings

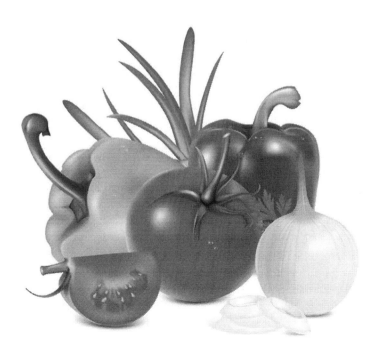

Pasta Salad

Ingredients

- 1 pound uncooked pasta

- 1 carrot, shredded

- 1 green pepper, seeded and chopped

- ½ cucumber, peeled and diced

- ½ onion, chopped

- 1 garlic clove, peeled and minced

- ¼ cup sun-dried tomatoes, chopped

- ½ cup vegetarian ham, cubed

- ½ to ¾ cup of your favorite dressing

- ¼ cup vegan feta cheese (page 81 - optional)

Directions

1. Put a pot of water on your stovetop to boil

2. While you are waiting, begin shredding and chopping the carrot, green pepper, cucumber, onion, garlic, tomatoes, and ham

3. When the water reaches a boil, pour in the pasta and cook according to the package directions

4. Once fully cooked, drained the pasta

5. Now pour the pasta into a medium-sized bowl

6. Add the ingredients you chopped and shredded and mix thoroughly

7. Add your favorite dressing and top with vegan feta cheese if desired

Makes 4 to 6 servings

Stuffed Mushrooms

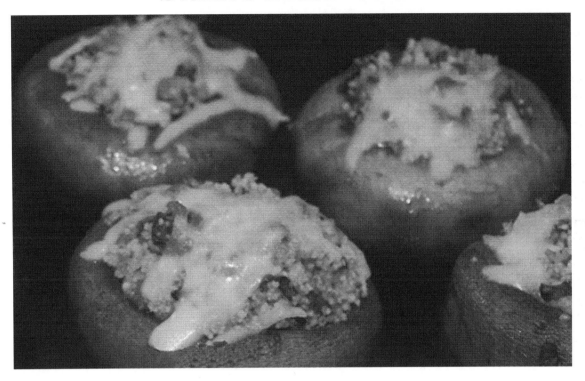

The stuffing for these mushrooms is so good. Just find any large open-cap mushroom to hold the filling and you'll find this recipe will become one of your favorites!

Ingredients

- 8 large open-cap mushrooms

- 1 tablespoon coconut or olive oil

- 1 small onion, peeled and chopped

- 2 garlic cloves, peeled and minced

- 1 stalk celery, chopped

- 1 carrot, peeled and chopped

- 1 zucchini, peeled and chopped

- 4 ounces extra-firm tofu, drained and diced

- 1/8 cup tomato paste

- 2 tablespoons fresh basil, chopped

- 1 teaspoon salt

- ½ teaspoon pepper

- 2 tablespoons pine nuts

- 6 ounces vegan shredded cheese (your choice)

- ¾ cup vegetable stock

Directions

1. Preheat your oven to 425 degrees F

2. Begin by washing the mushrooms and removing the stems from the caps

3. Take the stems and finely chop them

4. Using a large frying pan on your stovetop, heat up the oil

5. Once heated, add the onion, garlic, celery, carrot and zucchini to the pan

6. Sauté for 5 to 6 minutes until the vegetables are softened

7. Add the tofu, tomato paste, basil, salt, pepper, and pine nuts to the pan and cook for an additional 5 minutes

8. Remove from heat

9. Now evenly divide the stuffing mix from the frying pan into each mushroom cap

10. Place each stuffed cap into a shallow baking dish

11. Carefully sprinkle the shredded cheese on top of the mushrooms

12. Now pour the vegetable broth into the dish so it surrounds the mushrooms

13. Place baking dish into your preheated oven and cook for 20 to 25 minutes. Remove sooner if the cheese has melted and begins to turn brown

Makes 4 (2 mushrooms) servings

Jambalaya

Here is a colorful and nutritious way to enjoy a traditional favorite--only meatless!

Ingredients

- 2 tablespoons coconut or olive oil
- 1 onion, peeled and chopped
- 2 garlic cloves, peeled and minced
- 1 sweet bell pepper, seeded and diced
- 1 eggplant, peeled and diced
- 1 cup small broccoli floret pieces
- 6 baby ears of corn, cut in half lengthwise
- 2/3 cup frozen peas
- 1 cup tomatoes, diced
- ¾ cup vegetable broth
- 2 tablespoons tomato paste
- ½ teaspoon red pepper flakes
- 1 teaspoon salt
- ½ teaspoon pepper
- 1 teaspoon creole seasoning
- 2 cups brown or wild rice, cooked

Directions

1. In a large saucepan, heat up the oil
2. Once hot, add the onion, garlic, and pepper and sauté until the vegetables are tender
3. Add the eggplant, broccoli, corn, and peas until heated--about 5 minutes

4. Next, add in the diced tomatoes, vegetable broth, paste, pepper flakes, salt, pepper, and creole seasoning

5. Cover and cook over low heat for 20 to 25 minutes

6. Now add in the cooked rice and stir

7. Heat for an additional 3 to 5 minutes, then serve

Makes 4 servings

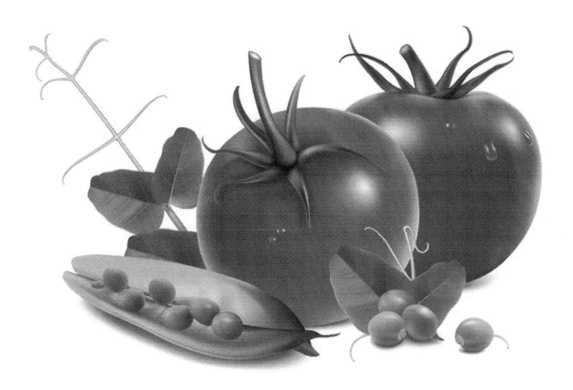

Dinner Recipes

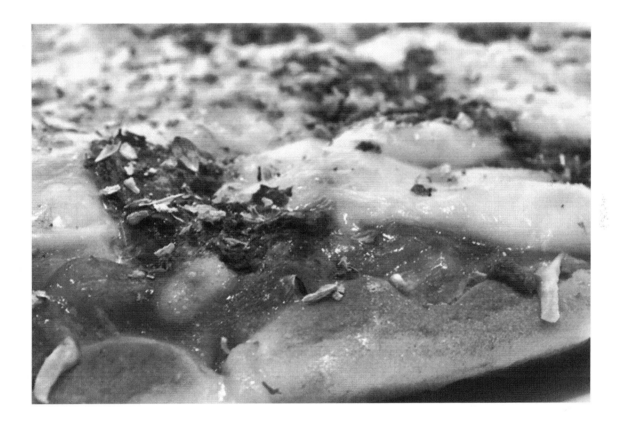

As a plant-based eater, you want your main dishes to be tasty and not difficult to make. With such busy schedules we all experience these days, I believe you will find these recipes easy to prepare with ingredients easy to obtain.

Eggplant Lasagna

Ingredients:

- 1 tablespoon coconut or olive oil

- 1 garlic clove, peeled and minced

- 1 small onion, peeled and chopped

- 1 eggplant, peeled and diced

- 1 (20 ounce) box or bag frozen spinach, defrosted and chopped

- 1 (64 ounce) jar pasta sauce

- 1 pound no-boil vegan lasagna noodles

Directions:

1. Preheat your oven to 375 degrees F

2. Take a medium skillet and make the oil hot

3. Sauté the garlic and onion for 3 to 4 minutes

4. Now add the eggplant and stir in with the garlic and onion

5. Place a cover over the skillet to allow the eggplant to become tender. This will take about 5 to 6 minutes

6. While the eggplant is cooking, lightly grease the bottom of a rectangular baking dish

7. Pour 2 cups of the pasta sauce on the bottom of the dish

8. Place 4 to 5 lasagna noodles over the pasta sauce

9. Place a thin layer of pasta sauce over the noodles

10. Follow this with a layer of the cooked eggplant

11. Now put another thin layer of pasta sauce on top of the eggplant

12. Add another layer of noodles

13. Put another thin layer of sauce, followed by the spinach

14. Continue in this way until the ingredients are used up

15. Cover the baking dish with aluminum foil

16. Place your baking dish in your preheated oven and bake for 45 to 50 minutes

17. Allow the lasagna to cool for 10 minutes

18. Cut and serve

Makes 6 to 8 servings

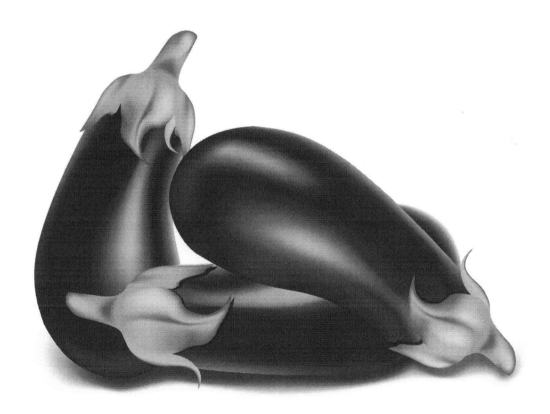

Fettuccine, Sprouts, and Cheese

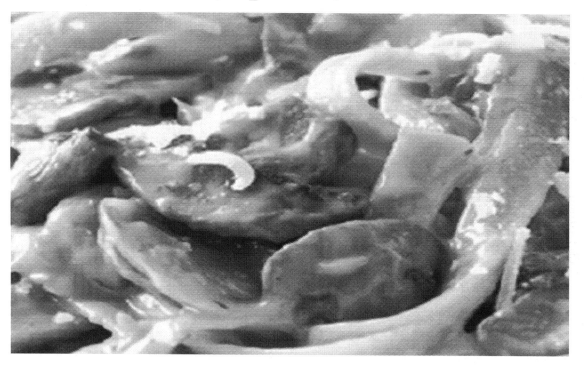

Ingredients:

- 1 (12 ounce) box fettuccine

- 1 tablespoon olive oil

- 4 cups Brussels sprouts, sliced

- 4 cups sliced mushrooms

- 2 garlic cloves, minced

- 2 tablespoons sherry vinegar

- 2 cups almond or coconut milk

- 2 tablespoons flour

- ½ teaspoon salt

- ½ teaspoon pepper

- 1 cup vegan Parmesan cheese (page 85)

Directions:

1. Begin by placing water in a large saucepan

2. Bring the water to boiling and place the pasta in the water

3. Boil for 10 minutes. Turn off heat

4. Drain and return the pasta to the pot with no heat

5. Take a large skillet and heat the oil over medium heat

6. Add the sprouts and mushrooms and cook for 10 minutes, stirring occasionally

7. Add the garlic and cook for additional minute

8. Add the sherry vinegar and continue cooking for another minute

9. Place the milk in a small bowl

10. Whisk the flour into the milk until the flour is dissolved

11. Now add the milk/flour mixture to the skillet

12. Season with the salt and pepper

13. Continue cooking and stirring until the sauce thickens. This should take just a few minutes

14. Add the cheese to the skillet until the cheese melts

15. Now add the sauce to the pasta in the pot

16. Toss gently and serve warmed

17. Feel free to top with additional cheese if desired

Makes 4 to 6 servings

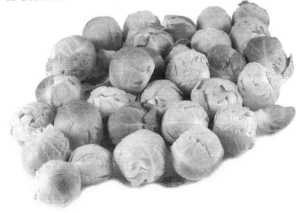

Coconut Polenta

Ingredients:

- 1 (28 ounce) can diced tomatoes

- ½ cup coconut milk

- 3 tablespoons coconut or olive oil

- 4 garlic cloves, diced

- 2 tablespoons of your favorite jerk seasoning

- 1 (15 ounce) can black beans, UNdrained

- 6 large stalks collard greens (Remove stems, then dice stems)

- 1 tablespoon apple cider vinegar

- ⅓ cup water

- 2 tablespoons chopped fresh thyme

- 1 (18 ounce) package polenta, precooked and sliced into ½ inch slices

Directions:

1. Preheat your oven to 350 degrees F

2. Lightly grease a rectangular baking dish

3. Add the entire can of tomatoes to the dish, along with the coconut milk

4. Place the dish into the oven and bake for 40 minutes

5. While things are cooking in the oven, place a skillet with 1 tablespoon of oil and heat over a medium setting

6. Add the garlic and jerk seasoning and cook until the garlic begins to brown

7. Now add the beans and turn heat down to low, stirring occasionally

8. Add the diced stems to the skillet and cook for 3 to 4 minutes

9. While the stems are softening, chop the collard leaves and add to the skillet

10. Add the vinegar and water to the skillet

11. Cover the skillet with a lid and lower the heat setting to low

12. After the tomatoes have finished cooking in the oven, add the thyme

13. In a separate skillet, add some more oil and heat over a medium setting

14. Place the polenta slices into the skillet and sprinkle with some additional jerk seasoning on each side as you cook it

15. Once the slices are browned, place a helping of collard greens over the slices, then topped with tomatoes

Makes 6 to 8 servings

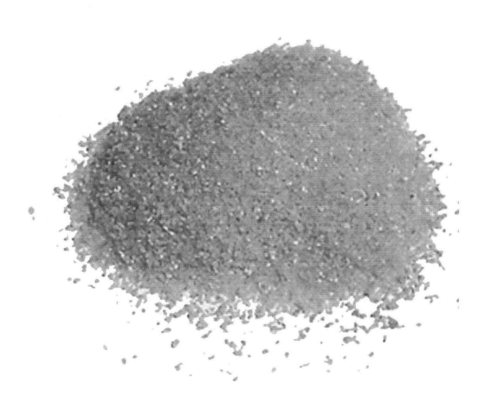

Homemade Pizza Dough

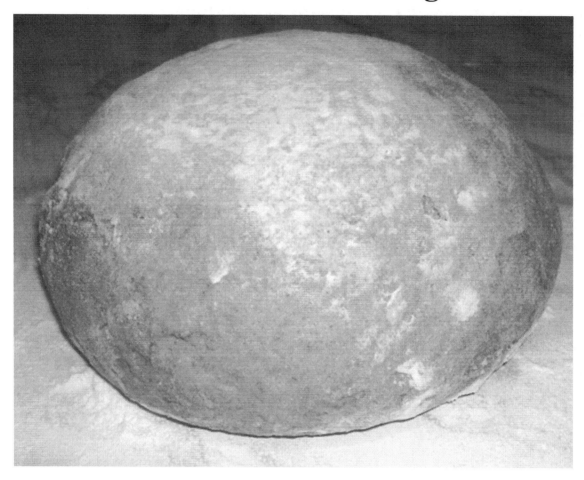

Here is a nice pizza dough that is vegan friendly. If you find that you like it, too, be sure to double the recipe and freeze half of the dough. It freezes well and is nice to have in reserve for the next time you want to enjoy homemade pizza.

For the preparation of this dough, you can either make it by hand or use a standing mixer.

Ingredients

- 1 cup warm water (just warmer than body temperature--about 105-110 degrees)

- 1 tablespoon instant yeast

- 1 tablespoon honey or sugar

- 3 cups unbleached bread flour (may need more for kneading)

- 1 teaspoon salt

- 1 tablespoon melted (not hot) coconut oil or olive oil

Directions

1. In a large bowl, add your warm water, yeast, and honey

2. Stir and allow it to process for 5 to 6 minutes

3. If bubbles and foam appear, your yeast is alive and effective. If no bubbles or foam appear, your yeast is dead and you will need new yeast.

4. Stir in approximately 2 cups of flour until thoroughly blended. (By hand, use a wooden spoon; by mixer, use dough hook)

5. Next sprinkle in the salt and mix until thoroughly blended

By hand:

- Add remaining flour using a wooden spoon

- When it gets too stiff to mix, it's time to use your hands

- Once 3 cups are worked into the dough, you will need to work the dough with your hands until the dough ball is not sticky any more and becomes elastic in consistency. It may be necessary to add small amounts of flour to the dough ball until it no longer sticks to your hands

- Work the dough ball for approximately 10 minutes to achieve this result

Note: If the dough ball seems too dry, drizzle a teaspoon of water or so into the dough and work it in

By mixer:

- Add in the third cup of flour and process on a lower speed

- After a minute, raise the speed to medium and allow the dough to be worked for approximately 5 minutes

- Now continue kneading the dough until it is smooth and has an elastic consistency. Add small amounts of flour if dough ball appears too sticky OR drizzle in small amounts of water (like 1 teaspoon) if the dough ball is too dry

1. Once you are satisfied with the consistency of the dough, remove it from the bowl to rest on an oiled section of your counter while you grease the bowl you were kneading in with some coconut oil or olive oil

2. Return the dough ball to the greased bowl

3. Now coat the top of the dough with oil as well

4. Cover the bowl with plastic wrap and then a dish towel

5. Allow the dough to rise in a warm place in your kitchen for approximately 60 to 90 minutes

6. The dough is ready when you use the flat, fleshy part of your finger to press into the dough and it leaves an impression

7. Using your fist, punch down the dough so the air bubbles are released

8. Work the dough again briefly to achieve a nice dough ball

9. You are now ready to make your pizza! Simply bake using your favorite recipe's instructions

Serving sizes:
- 2 (12-inch) pizza crusts

- 2 (9-inch) deep dish pizza crusts

- 4 to 6 (9-inch) pizza crusts

- 16 to 19 petite pizza crusts (size for an appetizer)

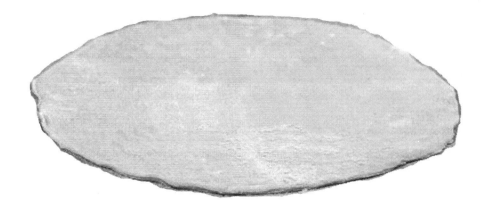

White Pizza

Here is a delicious recipe you can make using the Homemade Pizza Dough from the previous recipe.

Ingredients:

- 2 tablespoons olive oil

- 1 Homemade Pizza Dough ball OR 1 (24 ounces can Pillsbury® pizza dough)

- ¼ cup cornmeal

- 2 tablespoon Earth Balance Butter®

- 2 tablespoon flour

- 1 cup nut, rice or soy milk

- ½ teaspoon salt

- ⅛ teaspoon nutmeg

- ⅛ teaspoon cayenne

- 1 cup vegan Parmesan cheese (page 85)

- 1 pound asparagus, trimmed, cut into 2-inch pieces

- 4 ounces vegan shredded cheese (your choice)

Directions:

1. Preheat your oven to 450 degrees F

2. Lightly grease a large round pizza pan or a big cookie sheet

3. Lightly sprinkle the cornmeal over the oil

4. Now, spread your pizza dough out over the cornmeal and stretch it using either your hands or a rolling pin until it covers the pan. Now put the crust aside

5. Place a saucepan with water in it on the stovetop. This will be used to blanch the asparagus

6. While you are waiting for the water to boil, take a separate small saucepan and melt the butter over medium heat

7. Once the butter is melted, add the flour

8. Stir until the flour is dissolved and cook for 3 minutes

9. Now whisk in the milk and bring to a slow boil

10. Stirring occasionally, cook for 3 to 4 minutes, or until the sauce thickens

11. Now, turn off the heat and add in the salt, nutmeg, cayenne, and ½ cup of the Parmesan. (Save the rest for topping your pizza)

12. Now set this aside while you prepare the asparagus

13. Gently drop the asparagus pieces into the boiling water

14. Boil for 1 minute, then rinse the pieces with cold water to completely stop the cooking process

15. Drain

16. Now, return to your pizza dough and spread the white sauce over it evenly

17. Apply the cooled asparagus pieces all over the top of the white sauce

18. Sprinkle with the remaining Parmesan cheese and shredded cheese

19. Bake in your preheated oven for 20 minutes or until the top is browned and the crust is cooked completely.

Makes one large pizza

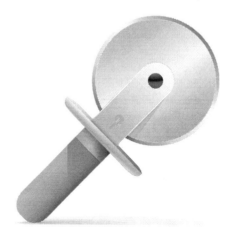

Pacific Tacos

Ingredients:

- 4½ tablespoons coconut oil

- 2 potatoes, peeled and cut in 1/2-inch cubes

- 1 cup corn (frozen or canned)

- 2 celery stalks, chopped

- 2 garlic cloves, chopped

- 1 bell pepper, chopped

- 1 onion, chopped

- Salt and pepper to taste

- Juice from 1 lime

- 10 corn tortillas

- 2 roasted chili peppers, chopped

- ¼ cup fresh cilantro

- Avocado slices

- Vegan shredded cheese and sour cream if desired

Directions:

1. Preheat your oven to 450 degrees F

2. Add 1 to 2 tablespoons of coconut oil to cover the bottom of a large skillet

3. Heat the oil and then add your potato slices

4. Fry the potatoes until they are golden brown and crispy

5. Drain the slices on paper towels when they are finished cooking

6. Add a little more oil to your skillet

7. Using a low heat, add the corn, celery, garlic, bell pepper, onion, salt, pepper, and lime juice

8. Cook for several minutes, stirring occasionally

9. Once the vegetables are tender and heated through, place them into a separate bowl

10. Now add the tortillas to your skillet, heating them up and gently frying them. This should be about 5 minutes on each side and should help soften them

11. To each tortilla, put some potatoes, followed by some chili peppers, cilantro, and the vegetable mixture you made

12. Finally, top with some avocado slices, shredded cheese and sour cream if desired

Makes 5 (2 tortilla) servings

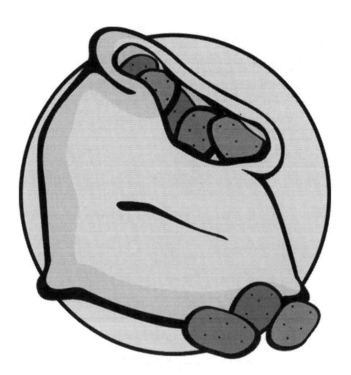

Veggie Pot Pies

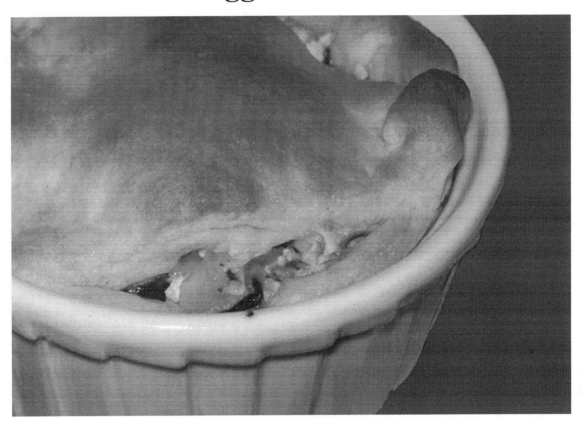

These cute little pot pies make just enough for a serving that is filling and tasty.

Ingredients:

- ¼ cup coconut oil

- 1 onion, chopped

- 1 large celery root, cubed

- 1 head of cauliflower, cut into small pieces

- 1 pound parsnips, cubed

- 1 pound Brussels sprouts, halved

- Salt and pepper to taste

- 1 teaspoon sage

- 1 teaspoon thyme

- 2½ cups almond milk

- 5 parsley sprigs

- ⅛ teaspoon dried sage

- ⅛ teaspoon dried thyme

- ½ onion, chopped

- 4 tablespoons Earth Balance Butter(R)

- ¼ cup flour

- ½ cup coconut milk (not light)

- ⅛ teaspoon nutmeg

- 1 (8 count) can Pillsbury Crescent Rolls® - original

Directions:

1. Preheat your oven to 375 degrees F

2. In a large frying pan, place your oil and heat until it is hot

3. Add in the onion, celery root, cauliflower, parsnip, and Brussels sprouts

4. Now add salt, pepper, sage and thyme to the vegetables and mix again

5. Cover and cook for about 30 minutes until the vegetables are tender

6. Remove the pan from the stovetop

7. In another saucepan, add the milk, parsley, sage, thyme, and onion

8. Do NOT heat. Simply cover the pan and allow the milk to sit for 20 minutes

9. In the meantime, take another saucepan over medium heat and melt the butter

10. Whisk in the flour and cook for 2 minutes, stirring constantly

11. From the saucepan you did not heat up, pour the milk mixture through a strainer and into the flour

12. Reduce the heat down to low and continue to whisk occasionally for 10 minutes. The mixture will be quite thick

13. Add the heavy cream and nutmeg along with any additional salt and pepper

14. Now add the sauce in together with the roasted vegetables

15. Place equal amounts of vegetable mixture into 8 lightly greased individual ceramic baking dishes—-about 4 inches in diameter (also known as ramekins)

16. Open the can of refrigerated crescent rolls and reshape the triangles gently so they are more rounded to fit on top of each dish

17. Place the dishes into a bigger baking dish that will hold all 8 ramekins and place this into your preheated oven for approximately 15 to 20 minutes—-until the crescent roll dough is golden brown and cooked through.

18. Remove from the oven and allow to cool briefly

Makes 8 servings

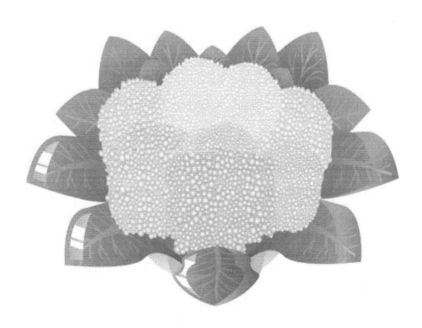

Grilled Tofu Kabobs

Ingredients:

- 1 (14 ounce) package extra-firm tofu

- 1 tablespoon tamari sauce

- 1 teaspoon ground ginger

- 1 tablespoon lime juice

- 16 cherry tomatoes

- 1 onion, peeled and quartered

- 1 bell pepper, cut into 1½ inch squares

- Oil for the grill

- ⅛ cup tamari sauce

- ⅛ cup molasses

Directions:

1. Drain the water from the tofu

2. Place a folded dish towel onto a cutting board or plate

3. Take a knife and cut the tofu horizontally in half. This results in two large slices that are about 1 inch in thickness

4. Set the tofu pieces on the dish towel

5. Place another folded dish towel on top of the tofu and put a heavy flat object on top-- an iron skillet or heavy pot will do nicely

6. Allow the weight to stay on the tofu for about 20 minutes

7. Once the object is removed, cut the tofu pieces so they are about 1½ inches squared

8. In a separate bowl, mix together the tamari sauce, ginger, and lime juice

9. Add the tofu pieces and toss until they are all coated

10. Cover the bowl and marinate in the refrigerator for 20 minutes

11. Now it's time to preheat your grill to a medium-high heat

12. Take grill skewers and begin threading the tofu, onions and peppers onto the skewers in alternating fashion

13. Mix together the tamari sauce and molasses in a small bowl

14. Using your grill tongs, take a folded paper towel and dip it into some oil

15. Rub the towel over your grill rack to create a non-stick coating

16. Place the kabobs on the grill for approximately 8 minutes, turning occasionally

17. Brush with the molasses/tamari mixture

18. The kabobs are done when the veggies are softened and the tofu is well glazed

19. Serve with your favorite side dish

Makes 4 servings

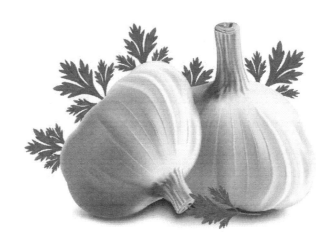

Fried Quesadillas

Ingredients:

- 1½ teaspoons tomato paste

- 1½ teaspoons apple cider vinegar

- ¼ cup barbecue sauce

- ⅛ teaspoon ground chipotle pepper

- 1 tablespoon olive oil

- ½ pound Portobello mushroom caps, diced

- ½ onion, diced

- 2 large whole-wheat tortillas

- ½ cup vegan shredded cheese (your choice)

Directions:

1. In a medium-sized bowl, combine the tomato paste, vinegar, barbecue sauce, and chipotle pepper and mix well

2. In a large frying pan, heat up 2 teaspoons of the oil over medium heat

3. Pour your mushrooms and onion into the frying pan and sauté for 5 to 6 minutes

4. After cooking, spoon the mushrooms into the barbecue mixture and mix well

5. Place the 2 tortillas on a plate or work surface

6. Sprinkle half of the shredded cheese on one side of each tortilla

7. Spoon some of the filling over the cheese

8. Now fold the tortilla over the filling and cheese

9. In your skillet, place another 2 teaspoons of oil in the pan and heat

10. Take your quesadilla and place it down into the oil and fry for 3 to 4 minutes, turning once

11. Remove from the pan and drain briefly on paper towels

12. Cut into wedges and serve with your favorite salsa

Makes 2 servings

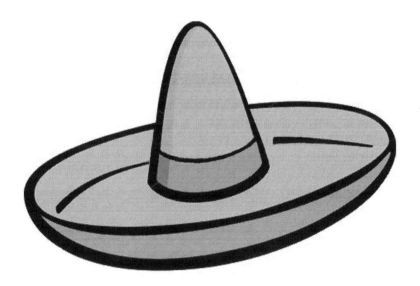

Veggie Burgers

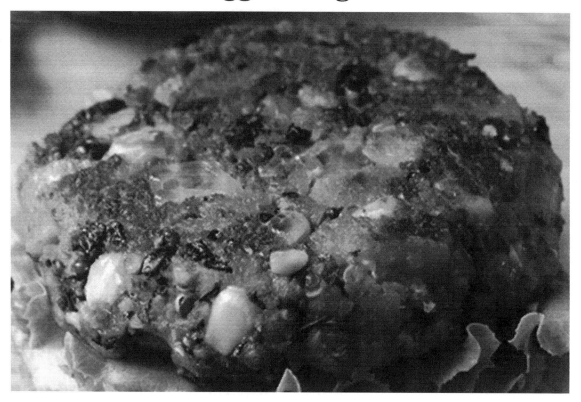

You can still enjoy a delicious burger with this recipe, plus you will get some healthy veggies included with this burger.

Ingredients:

- 3 tablespoons olive oil

- 8 mushrooms, diced

- 3 green onions, diced

- ½ bell pepper, diced

- ½ cup corn kernels

- 1 teaspoon cumin

- 2 garlic cloves, minced

- ¼ cup soft tofu

- 1 small potato, grated

- 1 carrot, grated

- Salt and pepper to taste

- ½ cup Panko bread crumbs

Directions:

1. In a large skillet, heat up the olive oil on your stovetop over medium heat

2. Add the mushrooms, green onions, bell pepper, and corn and cook them for 5 minutes

3. Now add the cumin and garlic and continue to cook for another minute or two

4. Remove from the heat

5. In a blender or food processor, process the tofu until you have a nice creamy consistency

6. In a medium-sized bowl, pour the creamy tofu, the mushroom and corn mixture from the skillet, as well as the potato, carrot, salt and pepper

7. Add the breadcrumbs and mix thoroughly until the mixture holds together. (Add additional bread crumbs if the mixture is too soupy)

8. After thoroughly blended, form the mixture into patties to the size you want and place them into the refrigerator for 2 hours

9. When ready to cook, place 2 tablespoons of oil into your skillet and heat it over medium heat

10. Once the oil is hot, carefully place the veggie patties into the oil and cook for approximately 3 to 4 minutes on each side

Spaghetti Squash with Avocados

Ingredients:

- 1 medium spaghetti squash

- 3 tablespoons olive oil

- 1 garlic clove, cut in half

- 2 avocados

- Juice from a fresh lemon

- 4 basil leaves, sliced

- ¼ cup vegan Parmesan cheese (page 85)

- 1 teaspoon pepper

- 1 teaspoon salt

Directions:

1. Preheat your oven to 375 degrees F

2. Using a heavy-duty knife, cut the squash lengthwise in half

3. Scrape out the seeds

4. Now lay the squash cut side down into a baking dish that can hold ¼ inch of water

5. Place in the oven and bake for 45 minutes. The inside should be tender

6. When the squash is 5 to 10 minutes from being done, put the oil into a skillet over low heat and add the garlic

7. Cook until you can begin to smell the garlic cooking. This will take just a few minutes and will flavor the oil

8. Remove the clove halves from the oil

9. Cut the avocados in half, remove the pit and peel

10. Squeeze the juice from the lemon over the halves of the avocados

11. When the squash is cooked, remove it from the oven and flip the halves over

12. Now use a fork to loosen the flesh from the skin. This creates the "spaghetti" for your dish

13. Place the spaghetti squash into a bowl, drizzle with the garlic-flavored oil, top with some avocado slices, Parmesan cheese, pepper and salt to taste

Makes 4 servings

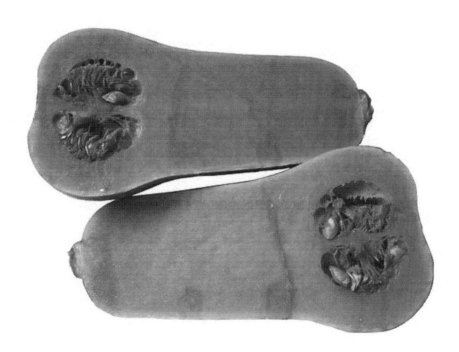

Lasagna Rollups

Ingredients:

- 4 sweet potatoes, cooked

- 4 cups fresh spinach

- 4 cups fresh basil leaves

- 5 garlic cloves

- 2 tablespoons olive oil

- ½ teaspoon salt

- ½ cup vegan Parmesan cheese (page 85)

- 1 (6 ounce) package vegan mozzarella cheese

- 15 ounces vegan ricotta cheese (page 109)

- Pepper to taste

- 2 cups marinara sauce

- 12 lasagna Dreamsfield® no-boil noodles

Directions:

1. Preheat your oven to 350 degrees F

2. Take your precooked sweet potatoes and remove the skins

3. Take a food processor or blender and put the spinach, basil, garlic, oil, and salt. This makes your pesto

4. Now add to the pesto the sweet potatoes, Parmesan cheese, ½ of the mozzarella cheese, and all the ricotta

5. Process all the ingredients until smooth

6. Season with additional salt and pepper if desired

7. Using a lightly greased 9" x 13" baking dish, spread about 1 cup of tomato sauce on the bottom of the dish

8. Take a lasagna noodle and spread some of the potato filling all over it

9. Starting at one end of the noodle, loosely roll it up

10. With the seam side down, place the rolled noodle into the baking dish with the tomato sauce

11. Repeat this process until all the noodles are filled and rolled

12. Place them snugly up against each other and top with the remaining tomato sauce

13. Cover the baking dish with foil and bake for 30 to 35 minutes

14. Now, remove the foil and sprinkle on the remaining mozzarella cheese

15. Place the dish back into the oven and finish cooking until the cheese browns

16. Allow to cool for 10 minutes once you remove the dish from the oven to let the rolls firm up

Makes 12 rollups

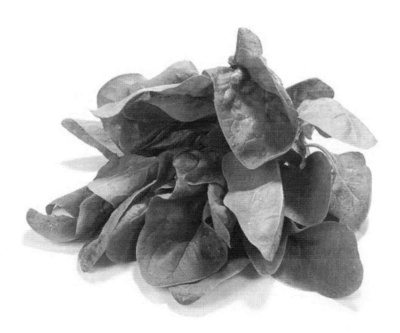

Bean Burritos

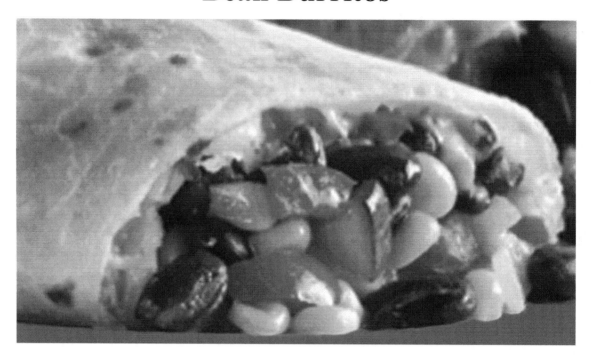

Ingredients:

- 1 tablespoon olive oil

- 1 garlic clove, minced

- ½ sweet bell pepper, seeded and diced

- ¼ teaspoon salt

- ½ teaspoon chili powder

- 1 zucchini, peeled and diced

- 1 (15-ounce) can kidney beans, drained

- 1 (15-ounce) can black beans, drained

- ⅓ cup water

- ¼ cup fresh salsa

- 8 large flour tortillas

- 4 Roma tomatoes, chopped
- 2 cups Romaine lettuce, shredded
- 6 green onions, chopped
- 6 ounces vegan shredded cheese (your choice)
- ¾ cup non-dairy sour cream

Directions:

1. In a large skillet, heat the oil over medium heat
2. Add the garlic and bell pepper and cook for approximately 2 minutes
3. Now stir in the salt, chili powder, zucchini, beans, water, and salsa
4. Reduce the heat and cook for about 10 minutes
5. Turn off the heat
6. Using a potato masher or fork, mash the bean mixture in the pan
7. Warm the tortillas by following the directions on the packaging
8. Once warmed, place the tortillas on serving plates and spoon an equal amount of the bean mixture into the center
9. Top the bean mixture with the tomatoes, lettuce, onion, cheese and sour cream
10. Roll up each tortilla and serve

Makes 8 servings

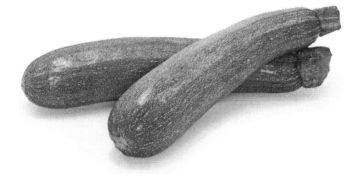

Curried Vegetables

Ingredients

- 2 tablespoons coconut oil or olive oil
- 1 onion, peeled and chopped
- 12 ounces red potatoes, cut into small cubes
- ½ head of cauliflower, broken into small florets
- 8 ounces turnips, cubes
- 2 garlic cloves, peeled and minced
- 2 teaspoons ground coriander
- 1 tablespoon fresh ginger, peeled and finely chopped
- 1 tablespoon curry powder
- 2 green chilies, seeded and chopped
- 1 tablespoon paprika
- 2 cups vegetable bouillon
- 1 eggplant, peeled and diced
- 1 (8 ounce) package mushrooms, buttons or thickly sliced
- 2 cups canned tomatoes
- 3 carrots, peeled and sliced
- 1 sweet bell pepper, seeded and sliced
- 2/3 cup coconut milk
- 1 tablespoon cornstarch
- ¼ cup chopped almonds

Directions

1. In a large cooking pot on your stovetop, heat up the coconut oil

2. When hot, add the onion, potato cubes, cauliflower, and turnip and cook for about 5 minutes

3. Now add in the garlic, coriander, ginger, curry powder, chilies, and paprika and stir together

4. Pour in the bouillon and stir it into the vegetables

5. Add the eggplant, mushrooms, canned tomatoes, carrot slices, and bell pepper

6. Place a cover on the pot and simmer on low for about 30 minutes to allow the vegetables to become tender

7. Stir the cornstarch into the coconut milk, making a smooth paste

8. Now stir the paste into the vegetables and combine thoroughly. This will thicken up the vegetable broth

9. Add the almonds and stir the contents of the pot constantly for 2 minutes.

10. Remove from heat

11. Serve over rice

Makes 4 to 5 servings

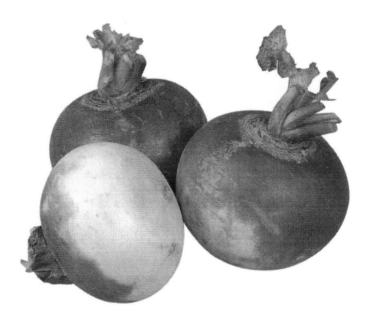

Potato Pan Pie

This dish offers a new presentation for a vegetable and potato meal.

Ingredients

- 1½ pounds red potatoes, sliced

- 3 cups small broccoli florets pieces

- 1 large carrot, peeled and diced

- ½ stick Earth Balance Butter®

- 2 tablespoons coconut oil

- 2 large garlic cloves, peeled and minced

- 1 medium red onion, peeled and cut into wedge slices

- ½ (12 ounce) package extra-firm tofu, drained and diced

- 2 tablespoons fresh sage, chopped

- 1 cup vegan cheddar cheese (page 112) or other non-dairy shredded cheese

Directions

1. In a large pot of boiling water on your stovetop, carefully pour in the potato slices and cook for 10 to 12 minutes

2. Drain to remove the water

3. In a second pot of boiling water, cook the broccoli pieces and carrot dices for 5 to 6 minutes

4. Drain to remove the water

5. In a large frying pan or skillet, heat up the butter and coconut oil

6. Once heated, add the garlic and onion and cook for 3 minutes

7. Now make a layer of potato slices on the bottom of the skillet using HALF of the slices

8. On top of the potato slices add the broccoli, carrots and tofu dices

9. Sprinkle 1 tablespoon of the fresh sage over the vegetables

10. Now place the other half of the potato slices on top of the vegetables

11. Sprinkle the cheese on top of the potato slices and continue to cook for 10 minutes

12. While the potato pie is cooking, turn on your broiler to preheat

13. After the 10 minutes, place the skillet under the broiler so the cheese will melt and turn brown

14. Remove the skillet from under the broiler and sprinkle on the remaining sage

15. Your dish is now ready to enjoy

Makes 4 to 5 servings

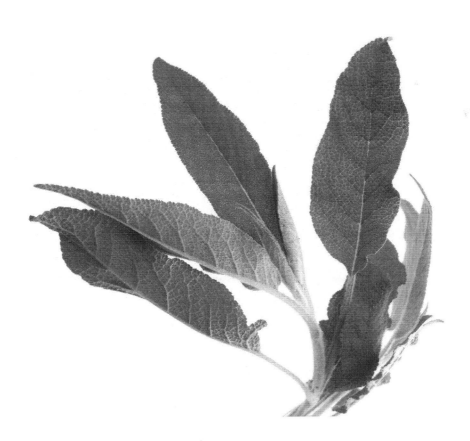

Black Bean Chili

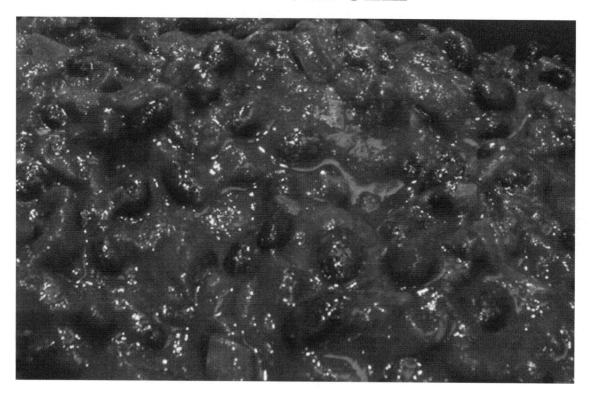

This chili recipe is so delicious. You won't want to miss out on this one and it's not hard to make at all!

Ingredients

- 1 tablespoon coconut oil

- 1 onion, peeled and diced

- 3 garlic cloves, peeled and minced

- 1 tablespoon salt

- 4 (15 ounce) cans black beans, drained

- 1 bunch cilantro, chopped

- 2 teaspoons cumin

- 1 teaspoon dried oregano

- 2 tablespoons dark chili powder

- 1 (28 ounce) can diced tomatoes

- 2 chipotle chilies in adobo sauce, chopped

- 2 tablespoons tomato paste

- 1 cup water

Directions

1. In a large pot on your stovetop, heat up the coconut oil

2. Add the onion and garlic and sauté until tender--about 5 minutes

3. Add the salt and beans to the pot and bring to a boil

4. Reduce the heat, cover the pot, and simmer 20 minutes

5. Add the cilantro and stir into the beans

6. Now add the cumin, oregano, and chili powder and stir it into the beans

7. Add in the diced tomatoes and chilies and cook for about 4 to 5 minutes

8. In a small bowl or cup, stir the tomato paste into the cup of water and then add to the beans

9. Continue to simmer over low heat for 10 to 15 more minutes

10. Serve and garnish with fresh cilantro if desired

Makes 6 to 8 servings

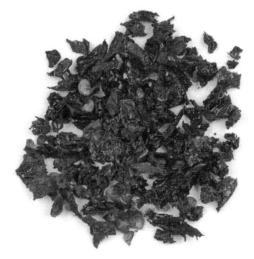

Fried Rice

Ingredients

- 3 tablespoons coconut oil

- 1 pound rice

- 1 onion, peeled and chopped

- 2 garlic cloves, peeled and minced

- 1 carrot, peeled and sliced

- 6 cups water

- 2 teaspoons salt

- ½ cup frozen green peas

- ½ cup frozen corn

- 4 green chilies, chopped

- 1 teaspoon ground cardamom

- 1 tablespoon dried coriander

- 1 tablespoon cumin seeds

- 2 crushed bay leaves

Directions

1. In a large pan, heat up the coconut oil over medium heat

2. Once the oil is hot, pour the rice into the oil

3. Sauté the rice until it begins to look golden brown

4. Add the onion and garlic and cook for another 4 minutes

5. Now add the carrot, water, salt, peas, corn, chilies, cardamom, coriander, cumin and bay leaves

6. Bring water to a boil

7. Now reduce the heat, cover the pot, and cook for 20 to 30 minutes--until the water is dissolved and the vegetables are tender

Makes 6 servings

Stuffed Crescent Rolls

Ingredients

- 1 tablespoon coconut or olive oil

- 1 onion, peeled and finely chopped

- 2 garlic cloves, peeled and minced

- 1 cup tiny pieces of broccoli florets

- 4 ounces mushrooms, finely chopped

- 2 (8 count) cans Pillsbury Crescent Rolls® - original

- ½ to ¾ cup vegan shredded cheese (your choice)

Directions

1. Preheat your oven to 350 degrees F

2. Lightly spray a cookie sheet with non-stick olive oil or coconut spray

3. On your stovetop in a medium frying pan, heat up the oil

4. Sauté the onion, garlic, broccoli, and mushrooms for 6 to 7 minutes--until vegetables are tender

5. Pop open the first of the two cans of crescent rolls

6. Separate the dough into 8 triangles

7. With a rolling pin or edge of a glass, gently roll the dough out some so it become slightly bigger than its original size

8. As you stretch each of the triangles, place them on your cookie sheet

9. Taking the vegetable mixture, equally divide it among the 8 triangles, placing the mixture in toward the center of each triangle so some edge is left for crimping

10. Sprinkle some of the shredded cheese on top of each triangle

11. Place one triangle on top of each triangle containing the stuffing so the edges match up with each other

12. Using a fork dipped in warm water, gently press the edges together (crimp) so the stuffing will be locked inside

13. Place in your preheated oven and bake for 18 to 20 minutes or until the crescent rolls are flaky and golden brown

Makes 8 servings

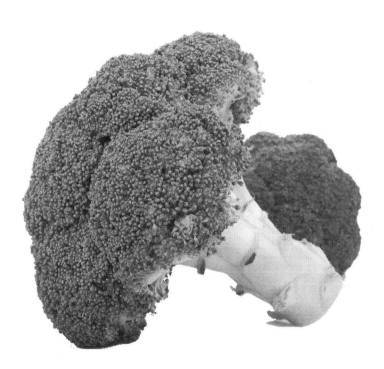

Vegetarian Sausage Loaf

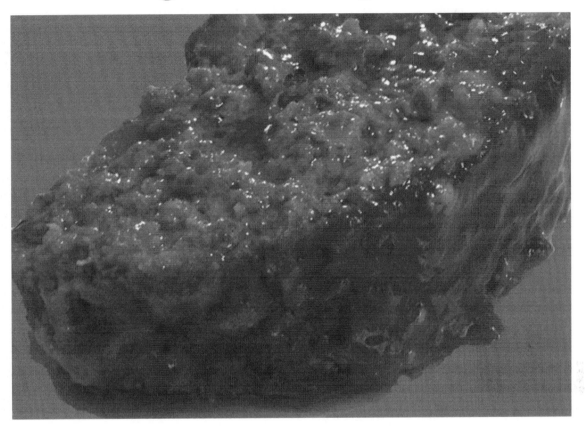

Ingredients

- 1 package medium-firm tofu (about 16 ounces)

- 1 sweet bell pepper, chopped

- 1 medium onion, chopped

- 2 garlic cloves, peeled and minced

- 1 vegetarian sausage (about 12 ounces), finely chopped

- 1 cup crumbled tortilla chips

- 1 teaspoon crushed espazote OR 1½ teaspoons dried cilantro

- 2 teaspoons salt

- 1 teaspoon coarse black pepper

- 2 cups of your favorite salsa

- 1 cup tomato sauce

- ½ to ¾ cup vegan shredded cheese (your choice of flavor)

Directions

1. Preheat your oven to 350 degrees F

2. Using a hand mixer, put the tofu, bell pepper, onion, garlic, sausage, chips, espazote, salt and pepper into a medium-sized mixing bowl and process on a medium speed

3. Mix until thoroughly blended

4. Treat a shallow baking dish with non-stick olive oil spray

5. Dump the loaf mixture into the baking dish and press firmly into a loaf

6. Place in your preheated oven and bake for 40 minutes

7. In a medium-sized bowl, mix the salsa and tomato sauce together until thoroughly blended

8. Remove the loaf from the oven briefly so you can apply the salsa/tomato mixture over the top of the loaf

9. Now sprinkle the cheese over the loaf

10. Place the loaf back into your oven and cook for an additional 10 to 15 minutes--until the cheese is melted

11. Allow the loaf to set for a few minutes before slicing

Makes 6 to 8 servings

Hearty and Spicy Soup

This delicious dish can be made on your stovetop using a cast-iron pot or Dutch oven. It cooks foods evenly and makes for an easy cleanup after dinner.

Ingredients

- 1 large onion, peeled and cut into wedges

- 1 cup chopped tomatoes

- 2 tablespoons spicy mustard

- 4 garlic cloves, peeled

- 2 teaspoons hot sauce

- 1 teaspoon soy sauce

- 1 tablespoon vinegar

- 2 teaspoons dried oregano

- ¼ teaspoon nutmeg

- 1 tablespoon smoked paprika

- 1 teaspoon thyme

- 1 teaspoon red pepper flakes

- 3 tablespoons coconut oil

- 2 tablespoons flour

- 8 ounces mushrooms

- 1 large zucchini, peeled and diced

- 2 cups sliced okra

- 1 (16 ounce) can black beans, drained

- 1 cup sliced celery

- 3 sweet bell peppers, seeded and diced

- 2½ cups vegetable broth
- 2 teaspoons salt

Directions

1. In a blender or food processor, combine the onion, tomatoes, mustard, garlic, hot sauce, soy sauce, vinegar, oregano, nutmeg, paprika, thyme, and red pepper flakes

2. Process until a smooth consistency is achieved

3. Set it aside for later

4. Place your pot on your stovetop and turn the heat to just below medium.

5. Heat up the oil

6. This next step will require your constant attention for 10 to 15 minutes: Now stir in the flour using a whisk to thoroughly combine the two

7. Continue to stir the mixture constantly over a low medium setting to allow a roux to be created and to keep it from burning.

8. Now pour the mixture from the blender or processor into the roux and mix thoroughly

9. Turn the heat up under the Dutch oven to medium and bring the mixture to a boil

10. Once a boil is reached, turn the heat back down to where it was

11. Add in the mushrooms, zucchini, okra, beans, celery, peppers, broth and salt

12. Place the cover on top of the oven and allow the vegetables to cook for 20 to 30 minutes

13. Once the vegetables are done, you are ready to serve up your soup

14. If desired, you can add in some cooked rice or serve the soup over rice

Makes 8 to 12 servings

Flavorful Couscous

With a dish like this one, you can serve it as a side dish or add your favorite meat substitute and make it a complete meal.

Ingredients:

- 1½ cups water

- ⅓ cup raisins

- 2 tablespoons coconut oil

- ½ teaspoon salt

- 1 cup couscous

- 1 onion, diced

- 2 garlic cloves, peeled and minced

- ⅓ cup toasted pine nuts

- 2 tablespoons capers, drained

- Salt and pepper to taste

Directions:

1. In a medium saucepan, bring the water, raisins, oil, and salt to a boil.

2. Once a boil is achieved, add the couscous.

3. Cover the pan and remove it from the heat.

4. Allow the mixture to stand for 20 minutes.

5. Take a skillet and place an additional tablespoon of oil in the pan and heat.

6. Once heated, add the onion and garlic and sauté until a golden brown.

7. After 20 minutes, fluff the couscous with a fork.

8. Now add the sautéed onions and garlic, the pine nuts, and capers.

9. Season with salt and pepper to taste.

Makes 4 to 6 servings

Enchiladas with Tofu

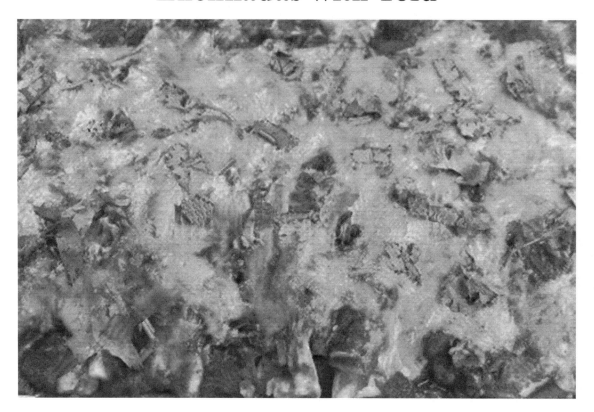

Ingredients

- 4-6 tablespoons coconut oil

- 1 small onion, peeled and chopped

- 6 garlic cloves, peeled and minced

- 1 small zucchini, peeled and chopped

- 1 small bell pepper, seeded and chopped

- 1 cup chopped mushrooms

- 2 jalapeños, seeded and chopped

- 2 limes

- 3 tablespoons pure maple syrup

- 1 package extra-firm tofu and cut into small cubes

- 1 teaspoon salt

- ½ teaspoon black pepper

- 1 tablespoon Mexican seasoning mix

- 12 corn tortillas

- 1 (8 ounce) package vegan shredded cheese (your choice)

- 1 (12 ounce) jar of enchilada sauce

- 1 (4 ounce) can green chilies (your choice of heat)

- 1 bunch fresh cilantro (chopped and used for garnish)

Directions:

1. Preheat your oven to 350 degrees F

2. Lightly grease a casserole dish with coconut oil

3. In a medium saucepan on your stovetop, heat up 2 tablespoons of coconut oil

4. Once heated, put in the onion and garlic

5. Sauté for 5 minutes

6. Now add the zucchini, bell pepper, mushrooms, and jalapenos

7. Continue to cook until tender and browned

8. Empty into a bowl and set aside

9. Now place 2 more tablespoons of coconut oil in your saucepan and heat up

10. Add the juice from 1 lime and the maple syrup and store

11. Add the tofu cubes and cook until the edges of the tofu begin to brown

12. Add the salt, pepper, and Mexican seasoning while the tofu is cooking

13. Once cooked, remove the pan from the heat and place in a separate bowl

14. Now that your filling is cooked, it is time to put the enchiladas together

15. Take each enchiladas, place a small amount of shredded cheese, a few tofu cubes, and about 1 tablespoon of vegetables

16. Roll up your tortilla and place it seam side down into your casserole dish

17. Continue in this manner until your filling is all used up. If you run out of tortilla first, just spread out the remaining ingredients on top of the enchiladas

18. Mix the enchilada sauce and green chilies together

19. Pour the sauce evenly over the enchiladas

20. Sprinkle your remaining shredded cheese over the top

21. Place the casserole dish into your preheated oven and bake for approximately 35 minutes

22. Once they are done, sprinkle the fresh cilantro over the top of your enchiladas

Makes 6 to 8 servings

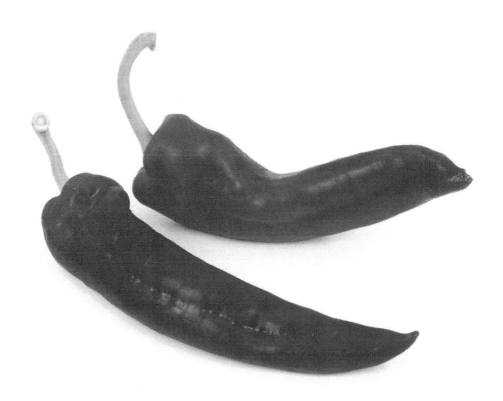

Creamy Chicken and Rice

Ingredients

- 1 tablespoon coconut oil

- 1 onion, peeled and chopped

- 1 (10 ounce) package chicken seitan strips

- ½ cup flour

- 1 (8 ounce) package mushrooms, sliced

- 1½ cups vegan chicken broth (Edwards & Sons Not Chicken Bouillon® is a good choice)

- 1 tablespoon soy sauce

- 2 cups favorite COOKED rice

- 1 teaspoon salt

- ½ teaspoon black pepper

- 1 cup milk alternative (almond, soy, etc.)

Directions

1. In a large saucepan on your stovetop, heat the oil

2. Once heated, add the onion and sauté until tender

3. While the onions are cooking, coat each seitan strip with the flour

4. Add each strip to the onions while they are cooking

5. Continue to cook the strips until they are nice and brown

6. Now add in the mushroom, cook for approximately 10 minutes and stir occasionally

7. Add in the chicken broth and soy sauce and stir gently

8. Then add the cooked rice, salt and pepper

9. Cover with a lid and lower the heat to simmer

10. Cook for approximately 10 minutes, allowing the mushrooms to become tender

11. Gently add in the milk and heat for a few more minutes--just enough to allow the milk to warm

Roasted Tofu

Ingredients:

- 1 (14 ounce) package extra-firm tofu

- 2 tablespoons balsamic vinegar

- 4 teaspoons coconut oil

- 2 tablespoons miso

- 1 pound asparagus, cut into 1-inch pieces

- 1 teaspoon orange zest

- 3 tablespoons fresh basil, chopped

- ¼ teaspoon salt

- ¼ cup orange juice

- 4 cups cooked rice or vegan noodles

Directions:

1. Preheat your oven to 450 degrees F

2. Take a cookie sheet and treat it with a non-stick cooking spray

3. Rinse the tofu and then pat it dry

4. Now cut the tofu into cubes, about ½ inch in size

5. In a large bowl, add 1 tablespoon of the vinegar, 2 teaspoons of the oil, and 1 tablespoon of the miso and mix

6. Place the tofu cubes into the bowl and coat with the mixture

7. Now spread the moistened tofu cubes onto the cookie sheet and place in the oven

8. Roast for approximately 20 minutes

9. Add the asparagus to the cookie sheet with the tofu and mix gently

10. Roast for an additional 10 minutes, allowing the asparagus to soften and the tofu to brown

11. While the cookie sheet is still in the oven, combine the remaining vinegar, oil, and miso together, along with the orange zest, basil, salt, and orange juice

12. Once the tofu and asparagus are done, spoon them into the bowl with the sauce and toss

13. Serve over rice or vegan noodles

Makes 4 servings

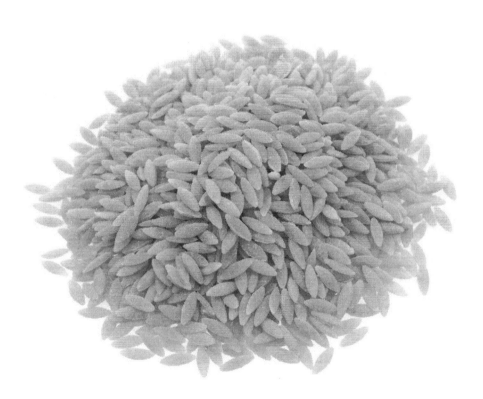

Peanut Soup

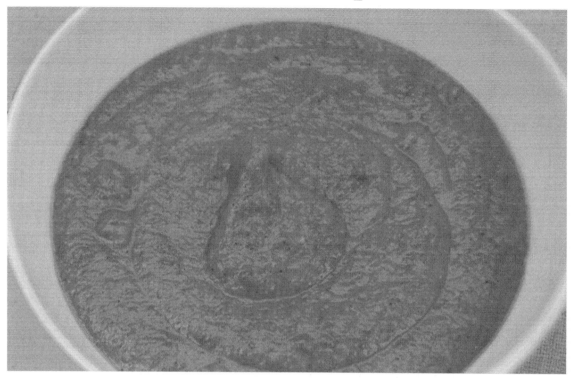

Ingredients

- 1 tablespoon coconut oil

- 1 carrot, peeled and grated (about 1/2 cup)

- 1 large onion, peeled and chopped

- 2 garlic cloves, peeled and minced

- 1 large sweet potato, peeled and grated

- 3 cups water

- ¼ teaspoon cayenne pepper

- 1 teaspoon curry powder

- ½ cup peanut butter

- 1 can condensed tomato soup (use an organic vegan one here)

- ½ cup non-dairy sour cream

Directions

1. In a large saucepan on your stovetop, heat the coconut oil

2. Add in the carrot pieces, onion and garlic and cook for approximately 5 minutes

3. Add in the grated sweet potato and water

4. Cover and simmer for 10 minutes--until the potato softens

5. Now add the cayenne pepper, curry powder, peanut butter, and condensed soup

6. Bring to a gentle boil

7. Remove from the heat

8. If you wish, you can make your soup a smoother consistency by using an immersion blender.

9. Just place it down inside your soup, turn it on, and blend until it is the consistency you like

10. Serve and top with sour cream if desired

To make this dish more like a complete meal, feel free to add your favorite meat substitute

Makes 4 servings

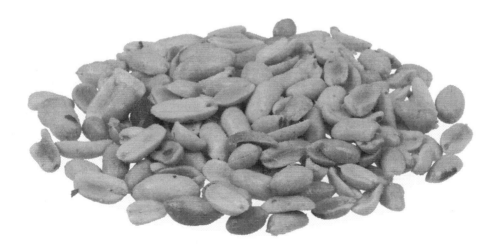

Creamy Tofu over Noodles

Ingredients

- 1 (12 ounce) package tofu, firm

- 3 tablespoons coconut oil

- 1 teaspoon salt

- ½ teaspoon pepper

- 1 (16 ounce) package sliced mushrooms

- 2 garlic cloves, peeled and minced

- 1 medium onion, peeled and chopped

- 1 tablespoon flour

- 1 tablespoon paprika

- ½ cup pineapple juice

- ¾ cup vegetable broth

- 2 tablespoons fresh tarragon, chopped

- 1 (8 ounce) package of your favorite vegan noodles

- 4 to 6 ounces non-dairy sour cream

Directions

1. Drain the tofu, then dice it into small cubes

2. Add 1 tablespoon coconut oil to a saucepan over medium heat

3. Once heated, add the tofu, salt, and pepper

4. Cook for 5 or 6 minutes until the tofu begins to brown

5. Remove tofu from the pan and set aside

6. Add 2 tablespoons coconut oil to the pan and heat

7. Add in the mushrooms, garlic and onion and sauté for 6 to 7 minutes

8. Add the tofu back in and combine

9. In a small dish, mix the flour and paprika together

10. Now sprinkle the flour/paprika mixture over the tofu and mix thoroughly

11. Add in the pineapple juice and cook until it becomes thicker

12. Gently pour in the vegetable broth

13. Cover the saucepan and turn your heat down to a low setting

14. Allow the tofu to cook for approximately 12 to 15 minutes, checking occasionally that it doesn't become dry. Add additional broth to allow a sauce to form

15. While the tofu is cooking, prepare your noodles according to the package directions

16. Sprinkle on the fresh tarragon when the sauce is done

17. Once the noodles are done, serve with tofu and top with sour cream if desired

Makes 4 servings

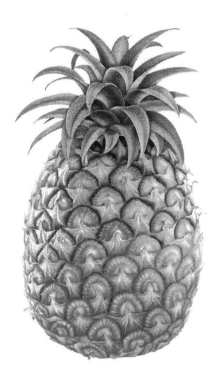

Black Beans and Rice Burritos

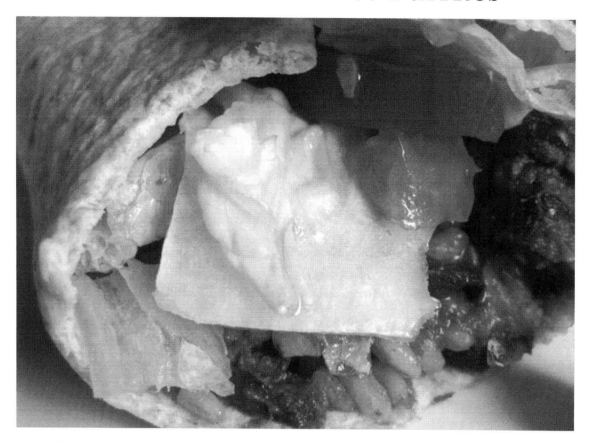

Ingredients

- ¼ cup of your favorite salsa

- 1 (15 ounce) can black beans, drained

- 1 cup brown rice, COOKED

- 4 (10-inch) flour tortillas

- 1 cup Romaine lettuce, shredded

- 1 large tomato, diced

- ½ cup non-dairy shredded cheese

Directions

1. Using a medium saucepan, place it over medium-low heat

2. Add in the salsa and beans and mix together

3. Add in the cooked rice and combine thoroughly

4. Heat for 4 to 5 minutes

5. Cover and remove from heat

6. In a large frying pan, heat up a tortilla so it is warm and pliable. (You can also do this in a microwave).

7. Place 1/4 of your bean mixture down the center of the tortilla, followed by some lettuce, tomato dices, and shredded cheese

8. Roll up the tortilla

9. Repeat this process for the other tortillas

Makes 4 servings

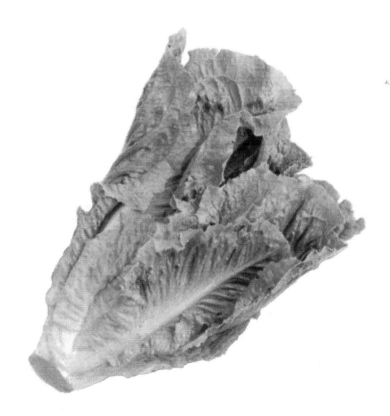

BLT's with a Twist

Ingredients

- 8-10 pieces of vegan bacon

- ½ cup vegan mayonnaise

- ½ teaspoon salt

- ¼ teaspoon black pepper

- 1/8 cup fresh basil, chopped

- 1 small lemon, zested

- 8 slices of bread (toast if desired)

- 1 large tomato, sliced

- 8 marinated artichoke hearts

- ¼ to ½ broccoli or alfalfa sprouts

Directions

1. In a medium to large frying pan on your stovetop, cook bacon until it is crispy, then drain

2. While the bacon is cooking, combine the mayonnaise, salt, pepper, basil, and lemon in a small bowl

3. Spread this mixture onto each slice of bread

4. Add the bacon slices onto 4 of the bread slices

5. Now top with a slice of tomato and artichoke heart slices

6. Add sprouts

7. Finish with the remaining slices of bread

Makes 4 sandwiches

Appetizer Recipes

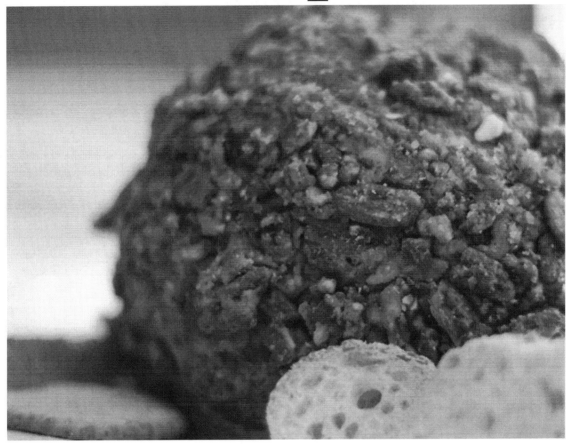

Delicious appetizers are not difficult to make at all, especially with all the non-dairy, egg-free, and milk alternatives available today. Whether you are having friends over, or you just want to pamper yourself and your family, you will find these recipes delicious and enjoyable to make.

Have fun!

Bacon Cheese Balls

This cheese ball will have your guests coming back for seconds, thirds, and fourths!

Ingredients:

- 2 (5 ounce) packages veggie bacon

- 1 green onion, chopped

- 2 (8 ounce) containers vegan cream cheese, softened

- 3 tablespoons vegan mayonnaise

- 1 cup chopped nuts

Directions:

1. In a large skillet, fry the veggie bacon

2. Allow the bacon to cool, and then crumble into small pieces or cut with a sharp knife

3. In a medium-sized bowl, put the bacon pieces, onion, cream cheese, and mayonnaise and mix thoroughly

4. Form into two equally-sized balls

5. Roll the balls into the chopped nuts, or refrigerate for several hours when the balls are firmer and roll in the nuts just before serving

6. Place in an air-tight container in your refrigerator until ready to eat

Makes 2 cheese balls

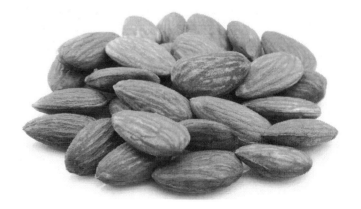

Fruity Salsa

Ingredients:

- 8 ounces raspberries

- 16 ounces strawberries

- 2 kiwis, peeled and diced

- 2 green apples, diced

- 3 tablespoons of your favorite fruit preserves

- 1 tablespoon brown sugar

- 2 tablespoons sugar

Directions:

1. In a bowl, put the raspberries, strawberries, kiwis, applies, fruit preserves, brown sugar, and white sugar and blend well.

2. Cover and place the fruit into the refrigerator and chill until ready to eat.

Makes 4 cups

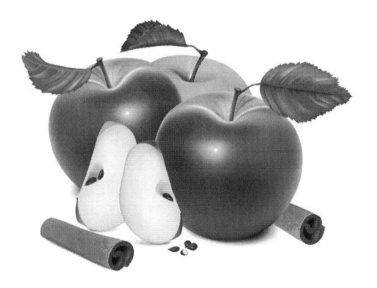

Mexican Layered Dip

Ingredients:

- 1 (16 ounce) can vegetarian refried beans

- 1 cup prepared guacamole (no gelatin added)

- 2 tablespoons taco seasoning mix (page 94)

- 1 (8 ounce) container non-dairy sour cream

- ¼ cup vegan mayonnaise

- 2 cups vegan shredded cheese (your choice)

- 1 large tomato, chopped

- ½ cup pickled jalapenos, sliced

- ¼ cup chopped green onions

- ¼ cup black olives, drained and chopped

- ¼ cup fresh cilantro, chopped

Directions:

1. Choose a pretty serving dish and spread the beans across the bottom

2. Next, spread the guacamole on top of the beans

3. Now mix up the seasoning mix with the sour cream and mayonnaise in a separate bowl

4. Spread this layer on top of the guacamole

5. Next, sprinkle a layer of cheese, followed by the chopped tomato, jalapenos, green onions, and olives

6. Sprinkle with fresh cilantro

7. Enjoy with a favorite cracker or chips

Note: If you wish, you can construct your dip on a pan that can go under your broiler. Then, when you have completed the layering, you can place it briefly under the broiler to melt the cheese. This dip is delicious when it is warmed up, too.

Colorful Bean Dip

Ingredients:

- 1 cup of your favorite salsa

- 1 (16 ounce) can vegetarian refried beans

- ½ teaspoon garlic powder

- 1 teaspoon ground cumin

- 2 tablespoons taco seasoning mix (page 94)

- 1 pint non-dairy sour cream

- 1 cup vegan shredded Monterey Jack cheese

- 2 cups vegan shredded Cheddar cheese

- 2 tomatoes, chopped

- 1 bunch green onions, chopped

Directions:

1. In a medium bowl, mix your salsa, beans, garlic powder, and cumin together thoroughly

2. Using a flat-bottomed serving dish, spread this mixture evenly on the bottom

3. Now mix the taco mix into the sour cream and spread over the beans as your next layer

4. Finally, sprinkle on the two kinds of cheeses, followed by the tomatoes and onions

5. This dip can be enjoyed with most any chip you like

Makes 4 cups

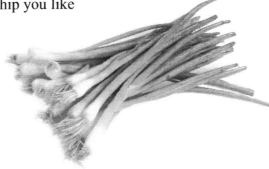

Veggie Bites

Ingredients:

- 1 can Pillsbury Crescent Rolls®

- 2 tablespoons dry Ranch-style dressing

- 1 (8 ounce) container non-dairy cream cheese, softened

- ½ cup chopped green bell pepper

- ½ cup chopped red bell peppers

- 2 carrots, finely chopped

- ½ cup chopped green onions

- ½ cup fresh broccoli, chopped

Directions:

1. Preheat your oven to 375 degrees F

2. Lightly grease a cookie sheet with non-stick cooking spray

3. Pop open the can of crescent rolls and place on the cookie sheet

4. Unroll the crescent rolls and form one big rectangular square. Pinch the seams back together along the perforated lines and stretch the dough out as much as you can without tearing it

5. Bake in your preheated oven for 10 to 12 minutes. You want the dough to be golden brown

6. Allow the dough to cool

7. In a medium bowl, mix the ranch dressing mix into the cream cheese

8. Once the dough is cool, spread this mixture over the dough

9. Now sprinkle and arrange the bell peppers, carrots, onions, and broccoli over the cream cheese mixture so they are evenly spread over the top

10. Chill in the refrigerator until completely cooled and slice into little bite-sized squares when ready to eat

Makes 6 to 8 servings

Marinated Veggies

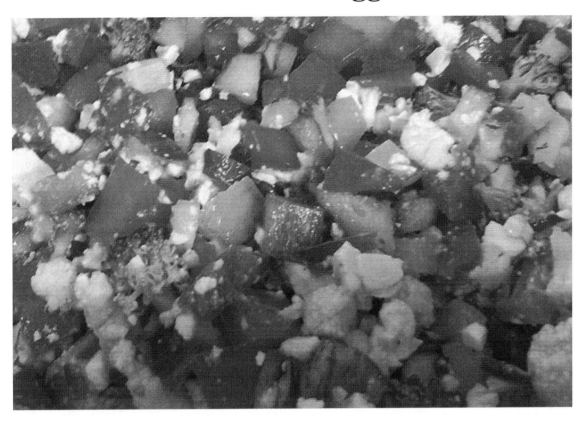

This is one of the prettiest dishes you will ever make. It is colorful, crunchy, and very tasty. Plus, it will feed numerous people. Consider this one for your next family and friend gathering.

Ingredients:

- 1 zucchini, diced

- 1 red bell pepper, diced

- 1 orange bell pepper, diced

- 1 yellow bell pepper, diced

- 1 yellow squash, diced

- 1 small red onion, diced

- 8 ounces mushrooms, sliced

- 16 cherry tomatoes, halved

- 1 cup broccoli, chopped

- 1 cup cauliflower, chopped

- ¾ cup cucumber, peeled and diced

- 2/3 cup olive or coconut oil

- 2/3 cup red wine vinegar

- 2 tablespoons sugar

- 2 teaspoons dry mustard

- 2 teaspoons salt

- 3 tablespoons dried parsley

- 3 garlic cloves, minced

Directions:

1. Start by placing the zucchini, bell peppers, squash, onion, mushrooms, tomatoes, broccoli, cauliflower, and cucumber into a large bowl and mixing them gently

2. In a small bowl, combine the oil, vinegar, sugar, mustard, salt, parsley, and garlic and mix thoroughly

3. Pour the oil/vinegar mixture over the fresh vegetables and mix thoroughly

4. Cover and place in your refrigerator to chill thoroughly before serving

Makes 6 to 8 servings

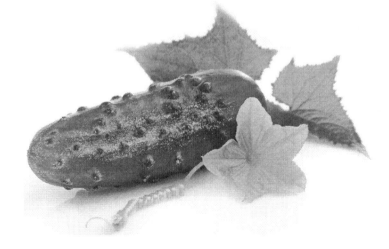

Potato Skins

Ingredients

- 4 baking potatoes, cooked and quartered

- ¼ cup non-dairy sour cream

- 2 tablespoons dry ranch dressing mix

- 1 cup vegan shredded cheddar cheese

- 1 bunch green onions, sliced

Directions

1. Preheat your oven to 375 degrees F

2. Scoop out the potato from the skins and place it in a bowl

3. Add in the sour cream and dressing mix

4. Using a hand mixer, combine the ingredient thoroughly

5. Fill the skins back up with the potato mixture and place on a baking sheet

6. Sprinkle the top with cheese

7. Place the baking sheet into your preheated oven

8. Bake for 12 to 15 minutes to allow the cheese to melt

9. Remove from the oven and sprinkle with the green onion slices

Makes 8 servings

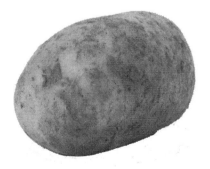

Pizza Rollups

Looking for a fun way to serve pizza? Here is a great solution. This is a great recipe to experiment with different ingredients for the filling, too.

Ingredients

- 1 (10 ounce) can Pillsbury Pizza Dough® OR make your own

- ½ cup vegan pizza sauce

- 24 slices vegan pepperoni

- 6 vegan string Mozzarella cheese sticks

Directions

1. Preheat your oven to 425 degrees F

2. Treat a baking sheet with non-stick cooking spray

3. Roll out your pizza dough onto the baking sheet so it is a large rectangle--about 9 inches x 12 inches

4. Cut the dough into 6 equal rectangles

5. Place about 1 tablespoon of pizza sauce on each rectangle and spread it out to cover the CENTER section of each one

6. Now place 4 pepperoni slices in the middle of each rectangle

7. Put a cheese stick on top next

8. Pull up each side of the rectangle over the cheese stick and pinch the ends to seal

9. Turn each rectangle over so the seams are down

10. Place the baking sheet into your preheated oven for 10 to 12 minutes or until the dough is golden brown

Makes 6 servings

Mushroom Ratatouille

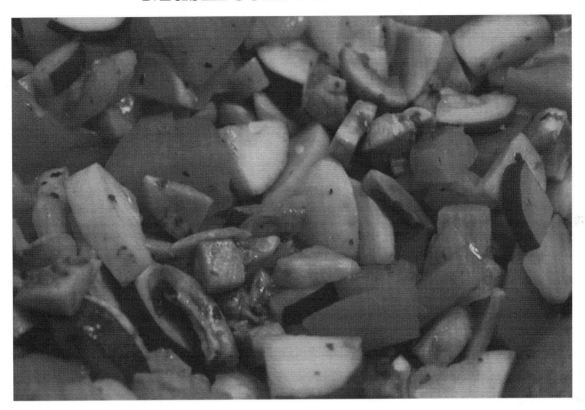

Ingredients

- 2 tablespoons coconut oil

- 4 garlic cloves, peeled and minced

- 1 large onion, peeled and chopped

- 1 (16 ounce) package mushrooms, chopped

- 1 cup vegetable broth

- 1 large tomato, chopped

- 2 tablespoons vegan Parmesan cheese (page 85)

- 2 tablespoons fresh parsley, chopped

- 3 (6-inch) pita breads

Directions

1. Preheat your broiler. You will be browning the pita bread slices under it later

2. On your stovetop, place a large skillet with the coconut oil in it

3. Once hot, sauté the garlic and onion

4. Now add the mushroom pieces and cook for 5 minutes

5. Gently pour in the vegetable broth and bring to a boil

6. Lower the heat but make sure the broth continues to boil and cook this way for approximately 10 minutes. The liquid should be absorbed by then

7. Turn off the heat

8. Add in the tomato, cheese, and parsley

9. Empty into a serving bowl

10. Take the pita bread and cut each one in half

11. Now stack the halves for each pita on top of each other

12. Make 3 equal triangular cuts, yielding 6 wedges for each pita

13. Arrange the wedges in a single layer on the baking sheet and place under the preheated broiler

14. Broil on each side to toast them

15. Allow them to cool off

16. When ready to serve, just spoon some ratatouille onto a wedge of toasted pita bread

Makes about 2 1/2 cups

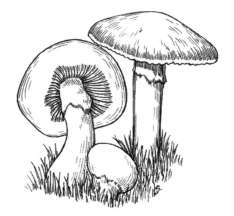

Cheesy Squares

Ingredients

- ¾ cup cornmeal

- 1¼ cups flour

- 4 teaspoons sugar

- 1 teaspoon Italian seasoning mix

- 2 teaspoons baking powder

- 2 green onions, sliced

- 1½ teaspoons Ener-G Egg Replacer®

- 2 tablespoons water

- ¼ cup coconut oil

- 1 cup milk alternative (nut, rice, soy, etc.)

- ½ green bell pepper, seeded and chopped

- ½ red bell pepper, seeded and chopped

- 4 ounces vegan shredded cheddar cheese

- ¼ cup cooked vegan bacon, crumbled

Directions

1. Preheat your oven to 400 degrees F

2. Treat an 11" x 7" baking dish with non-stick cooking spray or oil

3. In a large bowl, combine the cornmeal, flour, sugar, Italian mix, baking powder, and green onions together

4. In a separate bowl, combine the egg replacer with the water and stir until powder is dissolved

5. Add in the oil and milk and stir to mix

6. Now add the liquid to the dry ingredients and stir only until ingredients are moistened

7. Spread out the mixture evenly in your prepared baking dish

8. Sprinkle the bell peppers, cheese and crumbled bacon over the mixture

9. Place baking dish into preheated oven and bake for 25 to 30 minutes

10. Test for doneness using a toothpick or cake tester

11. Once finished cooking, remove from the oven and allow it to sit for about 10 minutes before serving

Makes 15 to 18 appetizers

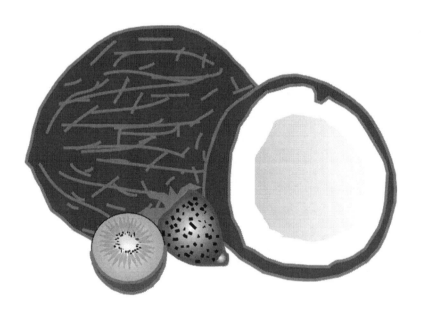

Delicious Wonton Bundles

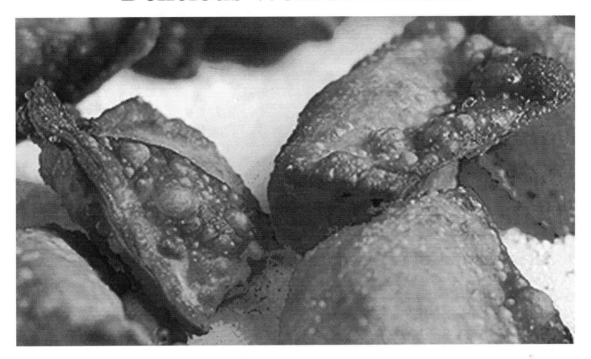

Crunch into these delicious bites of flavor and you will be the hit of the party, or evening, or whatever reason why you made them! Enjoy!

Ingredients:
Salsa

- 2 tablespoons coconut oil

- 1 (16 ounce) can whole tomatoes, undrained

- 2 garlic cloves, peeled and minced

- ½ onion, peeled and chopped

- 1 teaspoon salt

- 3 tablespoons fresh cilantro, chopped

Wonton Filling

- ½ pound vegan sausage

- 1 (4 ounce) can green chilies, chopped (heat of your choice)

- 1 cup vegan shredded cheese (your choice of flavors)

- 2 tablespoons green onion, chopped

- 40 eggless wonton wrappers

- 1 quart oil for frying

Directions

1. In a food processor, add the oil and undrained tomatoes and process until finely chopped

2. Pour into a saucepan

3. Add the garlic, onion, and salt and bring to a boil

4. Continue cooking for approximately 5 minutes

5. Remove from heat

6. Add chopped cilantro and set aside

7. In a skillet or frying pan, cook your sausage until browned

8. Drain if necessary

9. Place the sausage, chilies, cheese, and onion in a bowl and mix thoroughly

10. Take a wonton wrapper and place about a teaspoon of sausage mixture in the middle

11. Moisten two sides of the wonton with water using your fingertip

12. Fold the opposite sides of the wonton so they match up with the two sides you moistened

13. Gently squeeze out air as you pinch the edges together. You should now have a triangle

14. You can stop at this point if you want to, or moisten the two corners of the long side of the triangle and pinch them together with the third corner. It will look something like what is pictured at the top of the next page...

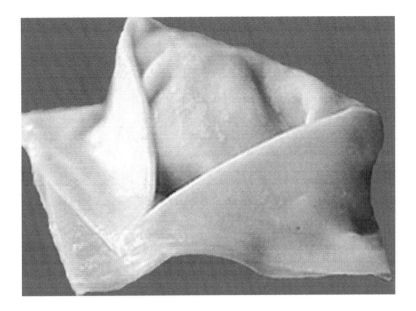

15. Continue in this fashion until all the wontons are filled

16. Heat up your oil in a 3-quart saucepan. If you have a deep fry thermometer, it should register around 365 degrees F

17. Gentle lower each bundle into the oil and cook for approximately 2 minutes each or until golden brown

18. Once cooked, drain on a paper towel

19. Serve with your salsa

Makes 40 wonton bundles

Spinach Stuffed Mushrooms

Ingredients

- 18 large button-shaped mushrooms

- 1 tablespoon coconut oil

- ½ onion, peeled and chopped

- 2 ounces pimento, drained and chopped

- 1 teaspoon lemon peel

- 1 tablespoon fresh lemon juice

- 1 (10 ounce) package frozen spinach, thawed and squeezed of excess liquid

Directions

1. Preheat your oven to 375 degrees F

2. Treat a 9" x 13" baking dish with non-stick cooking spray or oil

3. Remove the stems from the mushrooms

4. Using a damp paper towel, remove any dirt from the mushroom caps

5. Finely chop the stems of the mushrooms and set aside

6. On your stovetop, take a frying pan and place the oil in the pan and heat

7. Add the onion and chopped mushroom stems to the frying pan

8. Cook until the onions are soft

9. Now add in the pimiento, lemon peel, lemon juice, and spinach

10. Blend well

11. Remove from heat

12. Take each mushroom cap and fill it with the spinach stuffing

13. Now place each cap into your baking dish

14. Place the baking dish into your preheated oven and bake for 15 minutes

Makes 18 appetizers

Carrots with Pumpernickel

Ingredients

- 1 (8 ounce) container vegan cream cheese

- ½ teaspoon ground cinnamon

- 3 tablespoons orange juice concentrate

- ½ cup raisins

- ½ cup pecans, chopped (toast if desired)

- 1¼ cup carrot, shredded

- 1 package pumpernickel melba toast rounds

Directions

1. In a bowl, combine the cream cheese, cinnamon, and juice

2. Add in the raisins, pecans, and shredded carrot and combine well

3. Spoon about 1 tablespoon of this mixture on to the melba toast slices and eat

Makes about 15 to 18 servings

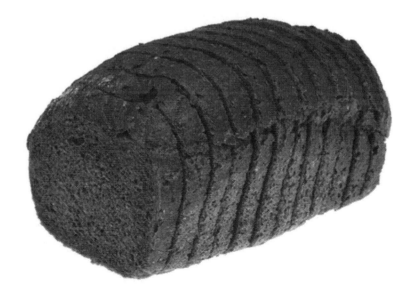

Quesadillas with Fruit

Ingredients

- 1 tablespoon lime juice

- 2 tablespoons fresh cilantro, chopped

- 1 (11 ounce) can mandarin oranges, drained and chopped

- 1/3 cup vegan feta cheese (page 81)

- 2/3 cup dates, finely chopped

- 2 tablespoons chopped green onion

- ¾ cup vegan shredded cheese (flavor of your choice)

- 4 (10 inch) tortillas

Directions

1. Preheat your oven to 375 degrees F

2. In a small bowl, combine the lime juice, cilantro, and drained oranges together

3. In another bowl, combine the feta cheese, dates, onion and shredded cheese together

4. Using a cookie sheet, place two tortillas beside each other on the sheet and put half of the salsa mixture and half the cheese mixture in the center of the tortillas

5. Using a pastry brush, moisten the outer edges of the tortillas with water

6. Place the other two tortillas on top and press down along the edges where you applied the water. This will help make a seal

7. Place the cookie sheet into your preheated oven and bake for 10 minutes

8. Cut the quesadillas into 6 to 8 wedges each

Makes 4 to 6 servings

Cheese Crackers

Ingredients

- ½ cup Earth Balance Butter®

- 3 tablespoons water

- 2 cups vegan shredded cheese (your choice of flavor)

- ½ cup vegan Parmesan cheese (page 85)

- ½ teaspoon salt

- 1 cup flour

- 2/3 cup sesame seeds

- 1 cup uncooked quick oats

Directions

1. In a mixing bowl, combine the butter, water, and cheeses with a hand mixer

2. Continue to mix while adding the salt, flour, sesame seeds and oats

3. Now shape the dough into a roll about 12 inches long

4. Wrap the roll in plastic wrap and refrigerate the dough for at least 5 hours

5. When it is time to bake the crackers, preheat your oven to 400 degrees F

6. Treat your cookie sheet with non-stick cooking spray or oil

7. Using dental floss, place the floss under the roll where you want to cut it, then criss-cross the floss as it cuts down into the dough

8. Continue to cut the dough into 1/4-inch slices and place the slices on your cookie sheet.

9. Place the cookie sheet into the oven and bake for approximately 10 minutes--until the edges are nice and brown

10. Remove from the oven and cool on a rack

Makes about 4 dozen crackers

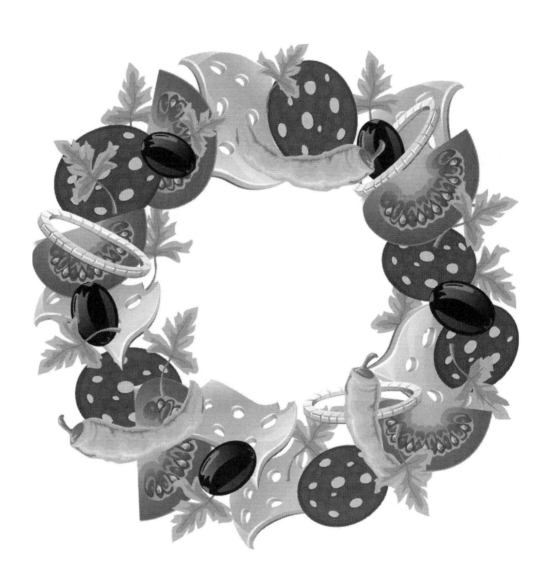

Appetizers

Dessert Recipes

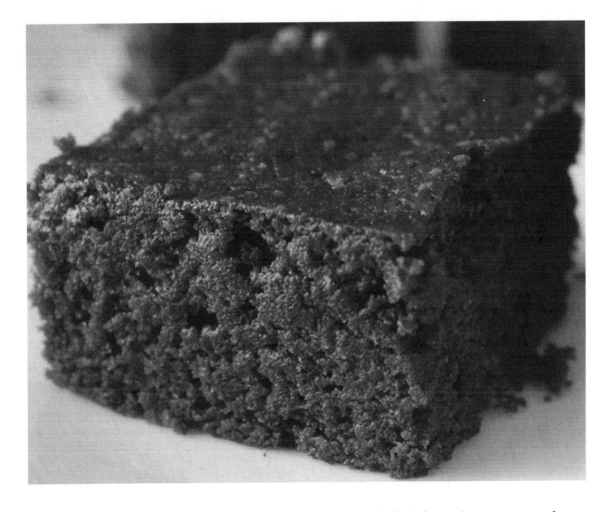

Just because you've chosen to eat a plant-based diet doesn't mean you have to miss out on dessert. You will see from this section that there are many delicious sweet treats you can enjoy and still stay true to your lifestyle.

Chocolate Cupcakes

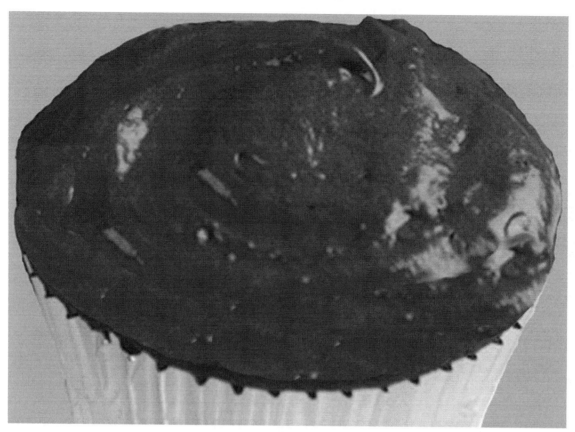

Ingredients
Cupcakes

- 1½ cups cocoa powder, unsweetened

- 1½ teaspoons baking soda

- 2 teaspoons baking powder

- 3 cups flour

- 1½ teaspoons salt

- 2 avocados, peeled and pitted

- 1½ cups milk alternative

- 2/3 cup coconut oil, melted

- 4 teaspoons pure vanilla extract

- 2 cups pure maple syrup

Frosting

- 3/8 cup pure maple syrup

- 1 teaspoon pure vanilla extract

- ½ block silken tofu, soft (drained and dried with paper towel)

- ¼ teaspoon salt

- 8 ounces vegan semisweet chocolate, melted

Directions

1. Preheat your oven to 350 degrees F

2. Take cupcake paper liners and place them into the muffin tins

3. In a large bowl, add the cocoa powder, baking soda, baking powder, flour and salt together thoroughly

4. In a blender or food processor, puree the avocados until smooth

5. Add in the milk, melted coconut oil, vanilla, and maple syrup and blend completely

6. Now add the liquids into the flour mixture and combine

7. Evenly divide the cupcake batter among the liners

8. Place the muffin tins into your preheated oven and bake for approximately 25 minutes

9. Test for doneness using a cake tester or toothpick

10. Cool on a wire rack completely

11. While the cupcakes are cooling, it's time to make the frosting

12. Using a blender or a food processor, combine the maple syrup, vanilla, tofu, and salt thoroughly

13. Add in the melted chocolate and blend until smooth

14. Pour the frosting into a bowl

15. Now dip the tops of your cooled cupcakes into the frosting, lifting each cupcake straight up out of the frosting, spin slightly and turn right side up

Makes 2 dozen cupcakes

Refreshing Fruity Pizza

Ingredients:

- ¼ cup confectioners' sugar

- 1 cup flour

- ½ cup Earth Balance Butter®

- 1/3 cup sugar

- 8 ounces non-dairy cream cheese

- 1 teaspoon vanilla extract

- 1 (11 ounce) can mandarin oranges, drained

- 2 cups fresh strawberries, sliced

- 1 cup fresh blueberries

Glaze

- 1 teaspoon lemon juice

- 5 teaspoons cornstarch

- 1¼ cups unsweetened pineapple juice

Directions:

1. Preheat your oven to 350 degrees F

2. Using a large bowl, combine the sugar and flour together

3. Cut in the butter until the flour mixture has a crumbly consistency

4. Using your hands, press this mixture out onto an ungreased 12-inch round pizza pan

5. Place in the preheated oven and bake for 11 to 12 minutes, or until the crust is lightly browned

6. Allow the crust to cool on a wire rack while you proceed with the toppings

7. In a small bowl, use a hand mixer to thoroughly blend the sugar, cream cheese, and vanilla

8. Spread this mixture evenly over your cooled pizza crust

9. Now arrange the oranges, strawberries, and blueberries to your liking over the pizza

10. To make the glaze, place a small saucepan on your stovetop and combine the lemon juice, cornstarch, and pineapple juice together

11. Bring to a boil and cook while stirring constantly for 2 minutes. This should result in the mixture thickening

12. Allow to cool for a few minutes, then pour the topping over the fruit

13. Place the entire pizza in your refrigerator and allow it to cool completely

Makes 1 (12-inch) pizza

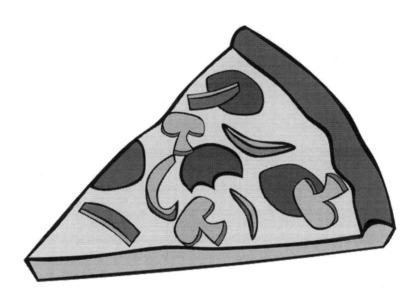

Gingerbread Cookies

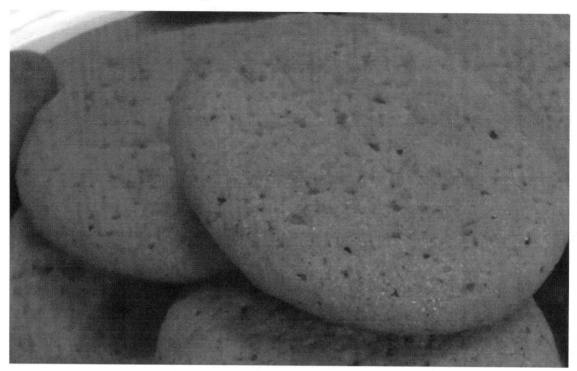

Ingredients:

- 1 cup sugar

- ¾ cup Earth Balance Butter®, softened

- ¼ cup dark molasses

- ⅓ cup water

- 1½ teaspoons baking soda

- ¼ teaspoon salt

- 2½ cups flour

- ½ teaspoon ground cloves

- 2 teaspoons ground ginger

- 1 teaspoon ground cinnamon

- ½ teaspoon nutmeg

- 2 tablespoons sugar

Directions:

1. Preheat your oven to 350 degrees F

2. Using a hand mixer and a large bowl, cream together the sugar and softened butter until the mixture is light and fluffy

3. Add the molasses and water and mix in

4. In a separate bowl, combine and whisk together the baking soda, salt, flour, cloves, ginger, cinnamon, and nutmeg

5. Now gradually add the dry ingredients to the butter mixture. Note: If the dough is too sticky, try adding a little additional flour so it can be handled and formed into balls.

6. Using an ungreased cookie sheet, scoop out a tablespoon's worth of dough and form into a ball and place onto the cookie sheet

7. Place the balls about 2 inches apart from each other on the sheet

8. Using a fork or your hand, flatten the balls slightly

9. Place in your preheated oven and bake for 12 to 15 minutes—until browned on the edges

10. Remove from the oven when browned and place on a cooling rack to cool

Makes 2 to 3 dozen cookies

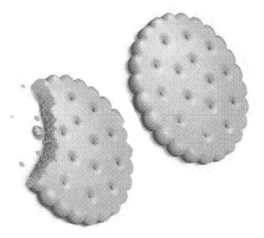

Nutty Chocolate Bars

Ingredients:

- 1½ cups peanut butter (smooth or crunchy)

- 3½ cups confectioners' sugar

- 1½ cups Nabisco Original Graham Cracker® crumbs

- 2 sticks of Earth Balance Butter®, melted

- 12 ounces vegan chocolate chips

Directions:

1. Using a medium-sized bowl, place the peanut butter, sugar, and cracker crumbs together and mix well

2. Once blended, add the melted butter and combine well

3. Lightly grease a 13 x 9 inch dish with a non-stick cooking spray

4. Now add the peanut butter mixture to the dish and spread out evenly

5. Using your microwave, put the chocolate chips into a microwavable bowl and process every 30 seconds, stirring each time, until the chips are a smooth consistency

6. Spread the chocolate over the peanut butter mixture

7. Allow the bars to harden either by refrigerating slightly, or allowing the chocolate to re-solidify at room temperature

8. Slice and enjoy

Makes 15-18 bars

Scrumptious Brownies

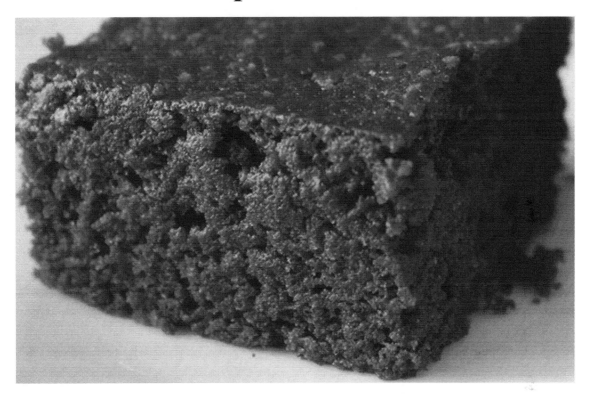

Ingredients:

- 2 sticks of Earth Balance Butter®, melted

- 1 cup unsweetened cocoa

- 2 cups sugar

- Equivalent of 4 eggs of Ener-G Egg Replacer®

- ½ teaspoon salt

- 4 teaspoons vanilla

- 1 cup all-purpose flour

- 4 cups vegan baking chips (one flavor or combination of several)

- 2 cups chopped nuts of your choice

Directions:

1. Preheat your oven to 350 degrees F

2. Grease a 9 x 13 inch baking dish with a non-stick cooking spray

3. Using a large bowl, combine the melted butter and cocoa and stir until the cocoa is thoroughly mixed in

4. Add the sugar and stir well

5. Add the egg replacer and stir until well blended

6. Now blend in the salt, vanilla, and flour until the flour just begins to disappear

7. Fold in the baking chips and nuts

8. Now spread the mixture in the pan and place in your preheated oven to bake for approximately 30 minutes

9. Cool completely before cutting into squares

Makes 15 to 18 brownies

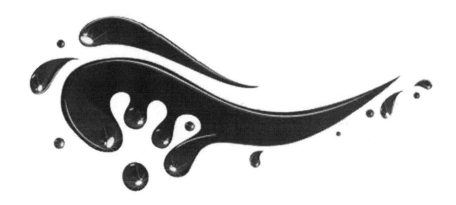

Pumpkin Cheesecake

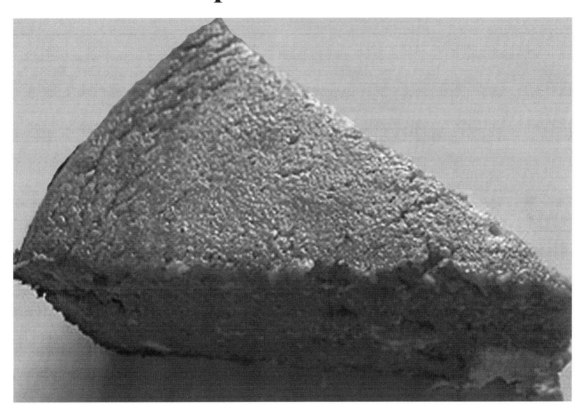

Ingredients

- 2 cups raw cashews

- 2 cups almonds, roasted

- 1 cup dates, pitted

- 2 cups 100% pumpkin puree

- ½ cup coconut oil, melted

- 3 tablespoons lemon juice

- ½ cup honey

- 4 teaspoons cinnamon

- 2 teaspoons ginger, ground

- 1 teaspoon nutmeg

- 1 teaspoon pure vanilla extract

Directions

1. Begin by soaking your raw cashews in water for 1 hour

2. Drain and set aside

3. Using a food processor, blend the almonds and dates until they are finely chopped

4. Lightly grease the bottom and sides of a 9-inch spring form pan

5. Press the almond/date mixture into the bottom of the pan

6. Wipe out your food processor with a paper towel

7. Now combine the pumpkin, oil, lemon juice, honey, cinnamon, ginger, nutmeg, and vanilla and process until the ingredients are creamy

8. Pour the pumpkin mixture into the spring-form pan and shake back and forth to smooth out the surface

9. Cover the pan with foil and place it into your freezer for 5 to 6 hours

10. Then transfer the cheesecake to your refrigerator an hour before serving

11. Remove the outer ring of the pan and serve

Makes 1 (9-inch) cheesecake

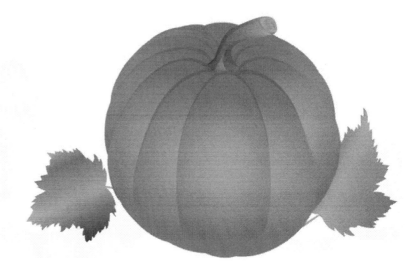

Incredibly Good Fudge

Ingredients

- 1 (16 ounce) non-dairy cream cheese

- 2 teaspoons pure vanilla extract

- 8 cups powdered sugar

- 2 cups non-dairy semisweet chocolate chips, melted

- 1 cup chopped nuts (optional)

Directions

1. Using a hand mixer, place the cream cheese into a large bowl and whip it until it is smooth

2. Now add in the vanilla and blend

3. Add in the powdered sugar a cup at a time and blend completely

4. Now place the chocolate chips in a microwavable bowl or you can put them into a double boiler.)

5. Process for 20 to 30 seconds each time, stir, and put back into your microwavable until the chips are completely melted and smooth

6. Now pour the chocolate into the cream cheese mixture and blend completely

7. Line a 9" x 9" pan with waxed paper or parchment paper

8. Pour the fudge liquid into the pan

9. Place in the refrigerator to firm it up

10. Once firm, remove the paper and cut into bite-sized pieces

11. Store in an airtight container in the refrigerator

Cherry Cobbler

Ingredients

Topping

- 2 cups walnuts

- 2 cups shredded coconut, unsweetened

- 2 teaspoons salt

- ½ cup Medjool dates, pitted

Filling

- 1 tablespoon lemon juice

- ½ cup dates, pitted

- 3 cups frozen cherries, thawed (be sure to drain, too)

- ¼ teaspoon ground cinnamon

Directions

1. To make the topping, pour the walnuts, coconut, and salt into a food processor and blend until smooth

2. Add 1 to 2 dates at a time and process. You want to have small crumbs when you are done

3. Set topping aside

4. To make the filling, place the lemon juice, dates, cherries, and cinnamon in a blender and process until you have a smooth consistency

5. Pour the cherry filling into an 8" x 8" square pan

6. Sprinkle the crumble topping over the cherry filling

7. Refrigerate and allow the cobbler to cool completely

Makes 3 to 4 servings

Lemon Bars

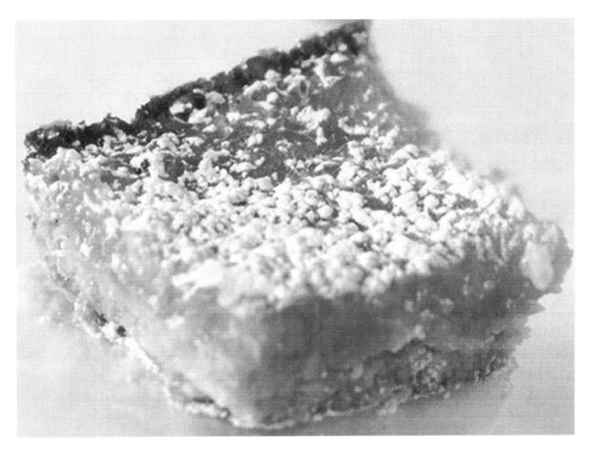

Ingredients

Crust

- ¼ cup confectioners' sugar
- ½ cup Earth Balance Butter®, room temperature
- 1 cup flour

Filling

- 2 tablespoons cornstarch
- 2 tablespoons flour
- ½ cup firm tofu
- 1 cup sugar

- 1/3 cup lemon juice, fresh squeezed (about 3 to 4 lemons)
- 3 tablespoons lemon zest

Directions

1. Preheat your oven to 350 degrees F

2. Treat an 8" x 8" baking dish with coconut oil or cooking spray

3. Sprinkle the bottom lightly with flour and discard any excess

4. Using a mixer, cream the sugar and butter together until light and fluffy

5. Now add in the flour and mix until a dough forms

6. Dump the dough into your baking dish and press it firmly into the bottom and out to the sides. Use the butter wrapping papers to make this job easier

7. Using a fork, make several holes in the top of the dough and place the dish into your preheated oven

8. Cook for approximately 20 minutes or until the crust achieves a nice golden brown color

9. Leave your oven on for when it comes time to bake the filling

10. Place the dish on a cooling rack while you start making your filling

11. Put the cornstarch and flour together in a small bowl and whisk together to combine

12. Set aside for now

13. Using your food processor or hand mixer, process the tofu until it becomes nice and creamy

14. Now add in the sugar and mix until the mixture becomes smooth

15. Add in the lemon juice, lemon zest, and flour until blend until thoroughly combined

16. Now pour your lemon filling into your cooled crust and place in your preheated oven

17. Bake for 30 to 40 minutes. You want the filling to become set. Although it may remain slightly giggly, it will set up more as it cools off

18. Place on a cooling rack and let it cool completely before serving

19. Optional confectioners' sugar may be sprinkled on after it is totally cooled

Makes 9 to 16 serving pieces

Layered Mousse Dessert

Ingredients

- 1 cup granulated sugar

- 2 (12.3 ounce) packages firm silken tofu

- 2 teaspoons pure vanilla extract

- 1 package vegan semisweet chocolate chips

- 2 tablespoons silk creamer

Directions

Note: You will be making two identical batches EXCEPT the second batch will be made without the chocolate chips

1. Using a food processor or hand mixer, put 1/2 cup of sugar along with 1 firm silken tofu package and 1 teaspoon vanilla in a bowl

2. Blend until completely smooth

3. Using your microwave or a double boiler, melt the chocolate chips so they are a smooth consistency

4. Add the chocolate to the tofu

5. Now slowly add in the silk creamer

6. Once you have a nice creamy mixture, set aside

7. Now repeat the same process but do so without adding any chocolate. This mixture will slightly runnier than the chocolate mixture

8. Using pretty glasses or bowl, begin alternating the chocolate and vanilla mixtures

9. Refrigerate and cool completely before serving

The Best Chocolate Chip Cookies

Ingredients

- ¼ cup sugar

- ¼ teaspoon baking soda

- ¼ cup potato starch flour

- ¼ cup brown rice flour

- ¼ cup tapioca starch flour

- ¼ cup sorghum flour

- ¼ teaspoon salt

- ¼ teaspoon xanthan gum

- 1/3 cup pure maple syrup

- ¼ cup coconut oil, melted but not hot

- 1½ teaspoons pure vanilla extract

- ¾ cup vegan semisweet chocolate chips

Directions

1. Preheat your oven to 350 degrees F

2. Line 1 or 2 cookie sheets with parchment paper. I find it's nice to use two cookie sheets, then I can get one ready while the other one cooks

3. In a medium-sized bowl, add the sugar, baking soda, potato flour, rice flour, tapioca flour, sorghum flour, salt, and xanthan gum

4. Stir to combine completely

5. Now using a hand mixer, add in the syrup, oil, and vanilla

6. By hand, fold in the chocolate chip and allow the dough to rest for 10 to 15 minutes. This will help thicken it before cooking

7. Drop about a tablespoon's worth of dough for each cookie onto the parchment paper, leaving a couple of inches between each one

8. Place the cookie sheet into your preheated oven and bake for approximately 10 minutes

9. Allow the cookies to cool on the sheet for 5 minutes--then remove to a cooling rack

Makes 1½ to 2 dozen cookies

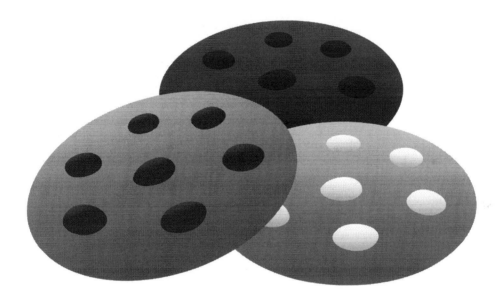

A Red Creamy Smoothie

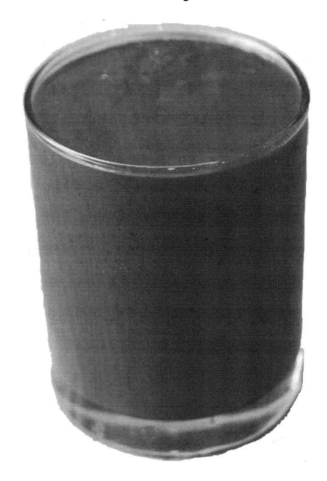

Ingredients

- 1 cup raspberries, frozen

- 1 cup coconut milk

- 1 very ripe banana (frozen if you desire a thicker and frothy smoothie)

- Juice from 1 lemon

- 1 tablespoon pure maple syrup or your favorite sweetener

Directions

Place all the ingredients into your blender and process until desired consistency

Makes 1 serving

Butter Pecan Ice Cream

Ingredients

- 3 tablespoons Earth Balance Butter®
- 1 cup chopped pecans
- 1 vanilla bean, split down the side lengthwise
- ½ cup sugar
- ½ teaspoon salt
- 2 (13.5 ounce) cans regular coconut milk (not low-fat)

Directions

1. In a small frying pan on your stove pan, melt 1 tablespoon of butter
2. Once heated, add the chopped pecans and cook for 3 to 4 minutes
3. Now transfer the pecans to a paper towel and allow them to drain and cool
4. In a medium saucepan on your stovetop, scrape the vanilla seeds from the bean
5. Add the sugar, salt, and coconut milk, and additional 2 tablespoons of butter and bring to a boil
6. Once a boil is reached, turn the flame down to low and simmer for 10 minutes, stirring occasionally
7. Now remove from heat, pour into a bowl and chill completely
8. Once the mixture is completely chilled, transfer to a blender and add 1/2 the pecans
9. Blend until the pecan pieces are quite small or until they are completely blended in with the coconut milk mixture
10. Pour the coconut milk mixture into an ice cream maker and process according to the maker's instructions (about 25 to 30 minutes)
11. Just before finishing, add in the additional pecan pieces
12. Serve immediately or place in a freezer-safe container to be enjoyed later

Makes about 1 quart

Delicious Homemade Candy

Ingredients

- 2 teaspoons pure vanilla extract

- 2 cups almond butter

- ½ teaspoon salt

- 1 cup water

- 2 cups sugar

- 2/3 cup corn syrup

- 1½ cups vegan semisweet chocolate chips

- 2 tablespoons coconut oil

Directions

1. Using coconut oil on a paper towel, lightly grease a 9" x 9" pan

2. In a medium saucepan on your stovetop, add the vanilla, almond butter, and salt

3. Over a low heat, heat up the contents, making sure not to burn it

4. Once heated, turn off heat but let the pan remain on the stovetop to keep contents warm

5. In another saucepan, combine the water, sugar, and corn syrup

6. Using a candy thermometer, heat until the temperature reaches 290 degrees F

7. Turn off heat and quickly add in the almond butter mixture

8. Pour into your prepared pan and spread out evenly

9. Place your pan on a cooling rack while you melt the chocolate

10. Using your microwave or double boiler, melt the chocolate chips

11. Once melted, add in the coconut oil and blend completely into the chocolate

12. Now pour the chocolate over the almond butter base and spread out evenly

13. Cool completely before slicing

Makes 16 to 25 pieces

Holiday Pumpkin Pie

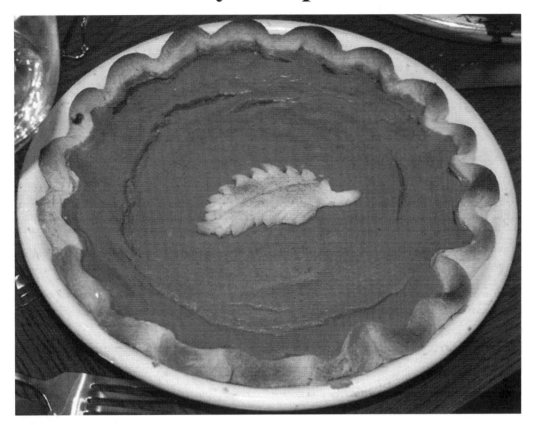

Ingredients
Crust

- ¾ teaspoon salt

- 1½ cups flour - don't pack firmly

- 3 tablespoons water

- 3/8 cup olive oil

Filling

- ¾ cup sugar

- 1 (13.5 ounce) can regular coconut milk (not low-fat)

- 2 cups 100% pumpkin puree

- 1 teaspoon cinnamon

- 1 teaspoon pure vanilla extract

- ½ teaspoon salt

- ½ teaspoon ground ginger

- ¼ teaspoon ground cloves

- ¼ cup corn starch

Directions

1. Preheat your oven to 350 degrees F

2. Cut two pieces of waxed paper for when it is time to roll out the dough

3. In a medium-sized bowl, add the salt and flour

4. Set aside

5. In a small mixing bowl, add the water and oil

6. Whisk quickly to combine them, then add them into the flour and salt

7. Combine just until the flour is moistened

8. Place your dough onto a sheet of waxed paper and place the second sheet on top

9. Using a rolling pin, roll the dough out until it will fit the size of your pie pan

10. Place dough inside pie pan and crimp the edges along the sides

11. Poke holes inside the bottom and along the sides of the pie crust with a fork

12. Place in your preheated oven and bake for 20 minutes

13. Remove from the oven and allow to cool while you make the filling

14. Turn the temperature of your oven up to 425 degrees F

15. Using a blender, add the sugar, milk, pumpkin, cinnamon, vanilla, salt, ginger, cloves and corn starch and process until smooth

16. Pour the mixture into your pie crust

17. Place in your preheated oven and bake for 15 to 20 minutes

18. Now lower the temperature to 350 degrees F and bake for an additional 50 to 55 minutes. You want the center of your pie to be set and not giggly

19. Remove from the oven and allow to cool on a wire rack

Makes 1 delicious pie!

Index of Main Recipe Ingredients

In this index, I have listed some of the main ingredients used in the recipes. If you are new to the plant-based lifestyle, this index will show you some of the ingredients that are often used in recipes. If you have been eating a plant-based diet for quite awhile, some of the ingredients listed in this index will be items you always keep on hand.

A list of spices, herbs and other condiments are listed beginning on page 22.

Under each item, I have included the page number to the recipe where that ingredient is used. I have also listed a few assorted topics covered in this book, along with their page numbers for easy reference.

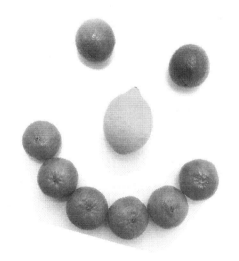

Additional Resources

Plant Based Nutrition: A Quick Start Guide for a Plant Based Diet

Plant Based Breakfast Recipes

Plant Based Lunch Recipes

Plant Based Dinner Recipes

Healthy Vegetarian Breakfasts

Healthy Vegetarian Lunches

Healthy Vegetarian Dinners

Healthy Vegetarian Collection

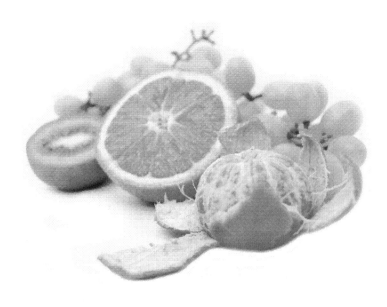

About Bindi Wetzel

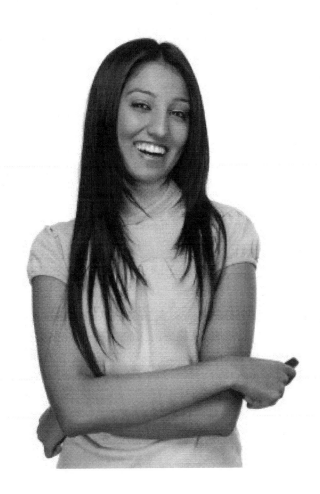

Bindi Wetzel is the author of the "Simply Vegetarian" cookbook series, a food writer, and teacher. She enjoys cooking simple dishes that are healthy and delicious.

Bindi dreams of one day opening her own vegetarian restaurant. Until then she experiments with creating new recipes that satisfy even the pickiest meat eater.

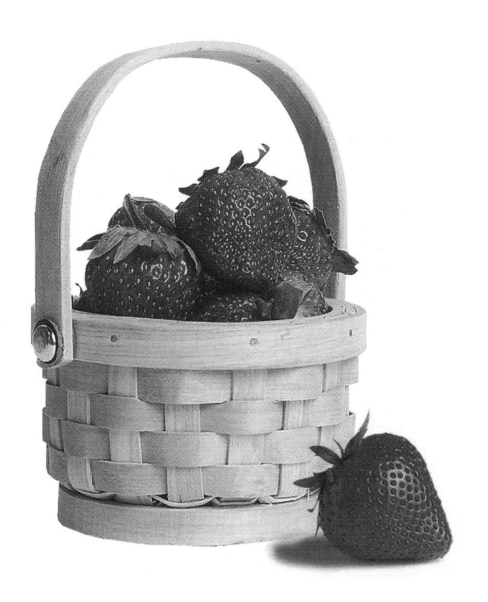

Made in the USA
San Bernardino, CA
25 July 2017